Daydreams & Diaries

By Taylor and Tim Black

D1570466

Untreed
Reads

Daydreams & Diaries
By Taylor and Tim Black

Copyright 2014 by Timothy W. Black
Cover Design by Ginny Glass

ISBN-13: 978-1-61187-388-7

Published by Untreed Reads, LLC
506 Kansas Street, San Francisco, CA 94107
http://www.untreedreads.com

Previously published in ebook:
Untreed Reads, 2011

Printed in the United States of America

"You don't get to choose how you're going to die or when. You can only decide how you're going to live."

Joan Baez quote found in Taylor's diary.

To Courtney, without whom this memoir would not have been possible.

CONTENTS

An Introduction

This is a story I hoped that I would never write and certainly when Taylor began her journey through brain cancer treatment we were both full of hope. After the shock of the initial experience and we realized that what always happened to others had happened to us, we still thought we would be different, that Taylor would be the one to beat the odds. It was that feeling that kept Taylor going and it was that hope that buoyed me up as well. Perhaps it was only denial, but that last year of her life is as vivid to me today, ten years later, as it was when it happened. Our hope was that something she and I wrote might help other young cancer patients cope with their disease and treatment. I still have that hope.

The memoir alternates between my fatherly recollections of my daughter throughout her life coupled with Taylor's actual diary (in italics) which she kept throughout her treatment. For the readers understanding, my daydreams of Taylor are also italicized, but actual conversations I had with her are in regular text.

Taylor kept a diary of her experiences from the day of her diagnosis until a few weeks before her death as CBS cameras followed her throughout that year as part of a *60 Minutes* program which would air, ironically, after her death, due to the events of September 11. The following excerpt if from her first diary entry when her journey began.

Taylor's Diary
September 23, 2000

I have just lived through the most indescribable night of my life. It all began when I was taking a shower on Thursday afternoon. My vision started to go in and out, I couldn't breathe. The next thing I know, I'm lying on the shower floor. I stood up and brushed it off as some fluke accident. For the rest of the day I was perfectly fine. And then, yesterday morning, my left leg became heavy and began to drag. Still, I thought nothing of it. So, naturally I thought Mom was going a bit overboard when she insisted on taking me to the Emergency Room. There I was, extremely frustrated, wasting a perfectly good Friday night in a hospital waiting room. Finally, they got me in and took a bunch of tests and did a CT scan.

When the doctor returned he looked visibly shaken. He approached us as if we were porcelain dolls, whispering something about a mass on my brain. All of a sudden I was whisked away in a wheelchair. As I looked down at the chart that I held in my hands I couldn't believe what was written there. Diagnosis: brain tumor. This can't be me, things like this happen to other people. People I don't know.

And so I settled into my hospital bed, too shocked to think. Then, Mom left to get my stuff (and freak out I'm sure) and I called Jeff to have him reassure me that this was a mistake. After I hung up on him, I called Katie to tell her that I was not going out with her tonight. Mom returned looking like she had been violently crying and bringing Chad with her. He assured me that everything was going to be alright and asked me if he should call my Dad. No way, that is just what I need on top of this mess: a dead father. Because if he were awoken at midnight and told that I have a brain tumor he surely would have a heart attack right then and there. No, I'll tell him tomorrow.

Taylor's Diary
September 28, 2000

These past few days have been a whirlwind. It feels like a haze has overcome me. Everyone is sending cards and calling. They look at me as if they have just run over my puppy. It is a look that reaffirms the magnitude of what is happening. Tomorrow I go in for brain surgery. I'm still waiting to wake up from the nightmare.

They are not sure what kind of tumor it is. So I'm spending the night before my surgery watching TV and talking on the phone. This can't be real! I have never, until last week, spent the night in a hospital and now I'm going for surgery tomorrow. Maybe after I do this then it will all turn out to be no big deal and everyone will feel stupid for getting so crazy over nothing.

The doctor claims he will cut as little hair as possible. I hope he is telling the truth. So, I have to go under the knife for 8 hours and then this will all be over. Well, that's not bad I guess. I suppose I should get some rest.

Chapter One: How Fathers Become Marshmallows

The memory is as vivid as the present…

Taylor is a few months old. She is bobbing atop our mercurial waterbed, cleaned and wiped with a fresh diaper that I have changed and I am alone with her in our bedroom.

I marvel at those big eyes. How did she ever get such big eyes? I lean over to sit beside her and cause the bed to jiggle. Taylor bobs a bit.

"Okay, Taylor, this is our bonding time, are you ready?" I ask.

Taylor doesn't respond. She doesn't understand a word I'm saying of course. So I decide to resort to song.

"I am going to sing you your grandfather Black's favorite song, *Red River Valley*, and then I will sing your Grandfather Joe's favorite, *Down in the Valley*. It seems your grandfathers were valley people, young lady."

As I begin to sing, I put a pinky finger in her little hand and she grabs on. I am bonding with my child. It is a wonderful feeling. The touch of the tiny, the innocent, the vulnerable, my blood. I begin to sing, *"From this valley they say you are going, I will miss your bright eyes and sweet smile…"* and Taylor begins to smile. My daughter appreciates good singing I think, either that or she is passing gas. I finish *Red River Valley* and begin *Down in the Valley* and Pam walks in.

"You know," she says. "Your daughter will someday fall in love with a cowboy because of this. She is going to love country music."

I smile at my wife. "Oh sure, right," I say.

But then I envision her as a young woman sitting in the audience at the Grand Old Opry in Nashville. That would be better than rock music, I think.

I sing *Red River Valley* another time, but this time cradling Taylor in my arms, kissing her lightly on the cheek. She gurgles and giggles. I'm hooked. My eyes moisten. I am so deeply in love with this baby girl. So small, so innocent, so alive.

And now just a memory.

Taylor's Diary
October 18, 2000

The doctor gave the news today with such a somber face,
They told me that they all would pray and leave me in God's
grace,
"We'll get through the weeks ahead, and you'll be fine I'm
sure," they said.
So much to take in such short time to have this happen in my
prime.
I really don't know what to feel, but everyone says it all will
heal.
If that is true and really is the case then why the sad look
upon your face?

Often Taylor preferred to write a poem about what she was going through rather than a straight narrative of her treatment.

Chapter Two: TV Star

I remember April of 2002. How could I ever forget? The hoopla of it all. My ex-wife Pam was excited about the CBS program *60 Minutes*. Both of the local newspapers—*The Palm Beach Post* and *The Stuart News*—ran articles about the local girl on the network program. *Desperately Fighting Cancer* the segment was billed.

Pam had a right to be excited I guess, although I was never a big believer in Taylor being part of that show, but then Henry Friedman at Duke University selected Taylor to be one of three brain cancer patients that CBS followed for months and I acquiesced, figuring that Taylor would get the best care possible if the cameras were rolling. "I think I can help somebody if I take part in the program," Taylor said. I still remember her saying that. Her motive was purer than mine. I wanted her to get the best possible medical care and she wanted to help someone else. And in the end she did. But not exactly how we thought she would.

As I turned the program on after the network tease with my deceased daughter, part of the promo of "a story you won't want to miss" or something like that, the choking in my throat began and the tears followed. Taylor had been dead for four months but there she was on the screen alive again in some surreal videotape with Pam and Courtney and the twins and Tracey Dawn at the hospital at Duke University. Only the CBS folks didn't tell the viewer that Taylor was dead, not until they pulled at the viewers' heartstrings with a double segment on (the damn thing would go on to win an Emmy for Ed Bradley, the only one of his career) Duke and the three patients they followed. It was all centered on the great man,

3

Henry Friedman M.D., who was Taylor's chief physician. A man whom Taylor liked and I didn't.

There were a few clips of Taylor at high school graduation receiving her diploma from the "Smiling Cobra" as teachers nicknamed Sara Wilcox, Superintendent of Schools. There was another clip of Taylor on the phone at her University of Central Florida apartment with the Friedmans (Henry the neuroncologist and Alan, the brain surgeon who would later work on Teddy Kennedy), yet another of Taylor getting the news that an experimental treatment didn't work, and Taylor acting stoically in an interview with Ed Bradley and responding to his question about her fear of death with a, "Yeah, I have thought about that, definitely. It's a very real possibility but everybody's got to die someday, and if I have to die, I have to die. I mean, I've come to grips with my own mortality now. Nobody lives forever. If I go a little bit earlier than I was—thought I was going to go—then I do, but at least make every day count, you know." To which Bradley replied, "You're amazing." I thought for a moment that Ed's earring might drop off and Taylor smiled sweetly with a big girlish giggle and responded, "Thank you." And Pam was all over the program which, of course, is fitting for a mother, but Pam's performance reminded me of a comment made about Teddy Roosevelt: "He wanted to be the bride at every wedding and the corpse at every funeral." But then again, Pam won three countywide elections for school board, which is a truly remarkable achievement. I ran once and got my clock cleaned. And she was incredible at Taylor's funeral when I couldn't say a thing.

Where was I on the show? Why wasn't I shown on the broadcast? It seems I was on the cutting room floor, a victim of an editor. The only *60 Minutes* interview I participated in was a taping at Duke that mercifully didn't make it into the broadcast. I was relieved. Taylor was telegenic. So were her sisters. So was Pam. I wasn't. Who wants a chubby old daddy on television? Maybe for a lousy sit-com with a laugh track, but not for prime time *60 Minutes*. Finally the agony of the segment was over. They cut to commercial.

And then Ed Bradley came back after the commercial for a "follow-up" at the end of the segment and told 20 million CBS viewers what I already knew, that shortly after filming that last segment of the experimental treatment at Duke, Taylor Black returned home to Stuart and died. Ironic now, when I think of it, that when he did that interview, Ed Bradley was suffering from cancer as well. I like to think that Taylor's courage might have influenced Ed Bradley. He sent me the nicest email about Taylor and it sits in the desk drawer with other Taylor memorabilia. I like to think that Taylor helped the CBS journalist in some small way for I was—and still am—Taylor's father after all and like so many other daddies, a daughter is my dawn, a sweet sunrise in every little smile. Thinking of the grin she gave Ed Bradley I truly know now the meaning of the word bittersweet; it was no longer just a word but a feeling that still courses through my body: bittersweet. There is an aftertaste of sorrow.

The program had been scheduled to air in the fall of 2001 but Osama bin Laden's attack on September 11th not only destroyed the twin towers and a piece of the Pentagon, but his perfidy threw a metaphorical monkey wrench into the

5

scheduled segments of *60 Minutes,* postponing Taylor's segments until the following spring. Oh, today the program is on the web, but I haven't been back to watch it in quite some time and I have a videotape copy as I never bothered to convert it to DVD since I never thought I would watch it again. I tucked a copy away in the desk in my den. Why should I watch Taylor in her last weeks, I don't need *60 Minutes* for that, for those days were permanently etched into my soul, a soul which was wounded when its sunshine was taken away.

In my mind the Carter Family is singing *You Are My Sunshine,* and I am rocking Taylor as a baby, singing along as I cradle her in my arms.

Taylor is alive again in my memory and, of course, on the internet for when I Google "Taylor Black Brain Cancer *60 Minutes,*" there she is once again "Desperately Fighting Cancer." Odd, as a history teacher, I think of the 19th century and the still photography. There is no doubt that the people in the photographs are indeed dead, unless of course, they are like the wizard photographs in the Harry Potter stories, where the characters in the photograph animate within the picture frame.

Taylor loved J.K. Rowling's work, but she didn't stay around to read all of the Potter novels for she had a prior appointment with her own form of Death Eater. But today, with the web, her images and sounds live on in cyberspace.

So Taylor was there, in the archives of *60 Minutes* and it was a wonderful program in its way but for Taylor *60 Minutes* was really only a Paul Harvey tease, for there was truly a "rest of the story."

Did *60 Minutes* explain the infinity symbol that she surreptitiously tattooed on her body at age 16 and which I didn't find out about until her cancer? Each of her six siblings and her sister-in-law and Melissa, the surrogate sister, had an infinity tattoo stitched on their bodies in remembrance of Taylor. Certainly Taylor's grit was apparent on the broadcast, but the CBS eye never captured her grace. I quibble I guess, but you can't reduce a life to a sound bite. Andy Warhol's famous phrase of "in the future everyone will be famous for fifteen minutes" was iconic, but it was also bullshit. He should have stuck to painting soup cans. Not everyone got their fifteen minutes, some got "60" but fame is a flicker, or in Elton John's words "a candle in the wind" and there was not one day in the past years that I wouldn't trade the hoopla of *60 Minutes* for a moment with Taylor.

Later, after the broadcast, Duke University reported a tremendous increase in inquiries about treatment for brain tumors; at the very least, the program helped someone, and Taylor would be happy with that.

Taylor's Diary
October 29, 2000

The anticipation of disease is a bitch no one should ever know.
The waiting is like a rollercoaster with the severest low.
Day in day out the same, no news has yet been heard,
And so the time will pass as we wait to learn the word.
A doctor here, a hospital there, to me it's all the same
For now I just sit waiting for the day that I go lame.
My body bruised and beaten will surely quit somehow,
Until that day, I'll wait and pray for when the time is now.

Chapter Three: Pot on Possum Long

I remembered all the concern about the year 2000. "Y-2K!" Everything was going to crash. For some reason, all of my life the year 2000 had contained a vague sense of foreboding for me. Call me crazy, and my ex-wife has, but even when I was young I had some strange fear of 2000 as if something bad were going to happen in that year. Superstition I guess, like the Mayans and 2012.

When Taylor and her girlfriend got "busted" for a joint of marijuana, I thought that was the seminal event of the year. Of course, I didn't know about it until big brother Chad clued me in as my ex-wife hadn't bothered to tell me of the arrest. Taylor had been at Pam's and while there she and a young lady—who shall not be named—were nabbed by the coppers with a bit of reefer. At one time or another some of Taylor's siblings had their share of "incidents" with the police, but Taylor was my only blood child who has entered the Miss Demeanor pageant. I found out when Taylor's hearing was and showed up at the courthouse. I said hello to Pam and she ignored me. Taylor, between us, rolled her eyes. Her parents exasperated her.

The judge gave Taylor probation and she was sufficiently contrite and I took her to a meeting of my 12-step program which was a joke as she had gone to the "Hall" for years for Thanksgiving and Christmas and knew quite a few of the people, but she said the Lord's prayer along with all of us and was polite to everyone. Yet she wasn't "one of us." In fact, she was a bit amused at me for dragging her there.

"Well, what do you think of the program, Taylor?" I asked her.

She smiled at me and replied with a touch of a mischievous twinkle in her eye. "I liked the prayer."

I couldn't help it, her comment made me laugh. I wasn't mad at her. I wasn't even disappointed. I was amused. But I was able to hide that…or at least I think I did.

Still I was irritated with Pam for not informing me of Taylor's bust but I was thankful she retained one of her former boyfriends as Taylor's attorney as he seemed to do a good job. I always admired her ability to get legal help. Later, Courtney told me the circumstances of the bust, or what I now refer to as the "Pot on Possum Long."

The girls parked across the street from the house of a police officer, who saw two girls smoking something suspicious in the car in the parking lot of the Possum Long Nature Trail where I had taken Taylor when she was a little girl and more interested in flowers than weed. Taylor was indeed culpable in the incident, but it was the other girl's grass and Taylor suggested that the other girl eat the stuff, but she didn't, and when the police officer knocked on the smoky car window and asked Taylor's buddy if they had anything, the girl had replied "weed" and Taylor took the blame because her buddy's mother was a total loon who would have freaked out on the other girl. Taylor got the probation and her pal didn't. Taylor "took the fall" for a friend, but she never told either Pam or I, only Courtney, and Courtney related that story to me after Taylor died, for it was a secret between sisters.

But then some odd karma took over I guess, for a few months later when Taylor was being treated for a brain tumor and being oh so politely poisoned by chemotherapy it was pot

10

and only pot that relieved the nausea of chemotherapy. All the wise solons in the U.S. Senate who are so opposed to medical use for marijuana should have to have a child with chemotherapy; they would change their tune then.

I guess "reefer madness" seems really inconsequential when you compare it to a brain tumor operation which would take Taylor and her family into uncharted territory. Taylor never tired of teasing me about her actually violating probation by using the marijuana during chemo. I wonder what she would say if she were here. Maybe…

Why not, Pops, you were the one who taught me about irony, always pointing it out in stories I read.

But you kids were really dumb to puff pot across the street from a police officer's house.

Can't argue that, Pops.

I don't know when I stopped being "Dad" and picked up the "Pops" moniker. When she was in tenth grade maybe? I said to Taylor in my mind,

Your Possum Long partner is out in Oregon now I think, finishing up her college degree.

She was on the eight-year college plan, Pops.

Why Oregon?

Why not?

Is it because of the pot laws?

Well, they don't hassle people for pot in Oregon.

That's why she went?

No, not really. Well, maybe. It's not like she is Polly Pot Head, Pops. Her grandparents are there and they volunteered to help her

pay for college if she came to Oregon. It's beautiful country out there, Pops.

You've been there?

Only when called, Pops, only when called.

Is Oregon like heaven?

No, Pops. Oregon is not like heaven. There is nothing like heaven on earth, but there is nothing like earth in heaven.

Chapter Four: The Elephant in the Living Room

I am reading from Taylor's diaries that Courtney found and shared with me. After discovering a poem I came across a statement she wrote: *So besides all that, mom's still an alcoholic, but I've decided not to deal with it.*

I'm glad you don't drink, Dad, Taylor's ten-year-old voice resonated in my head. I remember her saying that to me. She was little when I stopped drinking and didn't see me as the active alcoholic I once was. In fact, I might say that Courtney and Taylor inspired me to stay sober as I believed my daughters deserved a loving—and sober—father.

But her diary entry haunted me and took me back to a time that was most unpleasant for Taylor. One evening Taylor called me up to rescue her and I saw my ten-year-old daughter carrying her little Care Bear suitcase down Seashell Lane as I turned onto the street to scoop her up. She was crying and distraught and I would repeat that description in testimony the following year in a courtroom.

There would be many things the girls kept from me about their childhood on Seashell Lane, incidents that Courtney has related to me now, all those years later, which I am powerless to correct. I guess the girls were trying to protect the protector. I know now that their childhood was dysfunctional. And at one time I had been a part of that dysfunction.

In this family pot was not the drug of choice for substance abuse. Ours was a good middle class American family with its compliment of alcoholics, active and in recovery. After all, alcohol was legal and ours was a law and order family. Alcoholism is an insidious disease which still carries a stigma as if there was some moral failing in the suffering alcoholic, as if he just had some willpower he could stop drinking.

And for me alcoholism was progressive, if it wasn't arrested the disease just got worse. Where there were children involved there were safety issues. When my marriage began I had the problem, then we both had it, then I got much worse and was given my walking papers. Shortly after the divorce I got sober and remained that way.

Ironic, I suppose, but just like Jack Lemmon in the movie *The Days of Wine and Roses*, the separation saved my life, and the life of my daughters, for I entered my twelve step program and never left. One evening I would drive over and pick Taylor up, taking her out of an untenable situation.

I would go out and get a mortgage for a house which I allowed the girls to select in a neighborhood that was within a mile of mom's house so they could visit her on their bikes. Eventually the disease, and that's what alcoholism truly is, would take a sabbatical for a year or two in, shall I say, the Lee Remick character, with the benefit of some recovery before recurring in a bit milder form that Taylor was more able to deal with, as her later journal entry would suggest. But the elephant in the living room didn't go away entirely; in the year that Taylor was sick the elephant lurked and, on occasion, tromped around the living room.

I know the elephant was always lurking in me as well, only a drink away, but I was blessed by the fact that Taylor never saw me drink even if, over the years, I became something of an evangelist for temperance. Not surprisingly, some people didn't find my evangelism endearing.

As she entered adolescence, I realized Taylor was no little angel and that she drank as did nearly all of her peers. Like most parents, I didn't know to what extent my child drank. Certainly she didn't drink in my house, but I have a picture of Taylor with a beer bottle in her hand alongside her girlfriends at age 16 or 17. But there was no photo album of debauchery.

My own twelve step program was the equivalent of a crucifix to keep the disease at bay and the famous "steps" have been effective all these many years, but not everyone "gets it" and that is a shame for Taylor deserved better, every child deserves better and there was always a shadow of sadness on Taylor's face and in her big brown eyes turned inward when the subject of alcoholism was broached with her. It was her parents' Achilles Heel. I ached for Taylor, but I was unable to do anything to help her. I wondered if she picked up that beer in the photograph in a mimicry of someone she dearly loved but couldn't understand, for addiction is difficult to comprehend. That Taylor developed an Al-Anon approach was, I believe, the wisest thing she could have done. She and Courtney were the only kids among the seven siblings that took that approach initially.

I'm glad you never drink, Pops, she says to me now.

So am I Taylor, so am I.

How many years now, Pops?

Reagan was president when I last had a beer.

Gee, you're old, Pops. I see that pixie smile, which always accompanied her teasing.

Don't I know.

She used to say, *What's it like to be old, Pops?* That's one thing she'll never know. What it's like to be old. Growing old can be lonely, Taylor. It can be lonely. Until you show up and weave another dream for me.

Taylor's Diary
November 20, 2000

Today is the 20th anniversary of my elder sister Courtney's birth. And on this day that she is reflecting on her past as well as her future, I have taken the day to make light of the present events which are occurring. I have come to this conclusion: This is a magnificent experience which is putting forth. So I can uncover a secret to truly appreciate the beauty around me. The seriousness of the situation is awakening me and allowing me to live this beautiful life the way it was intended to be lived. I can feel the love and amazement penetrating my soul. Although my physical body is manifested with disease, my spiritual body is only now being cleansed. All the impurities that have before weathered my soul are now being washed away by the purest rain. I believe that when this experience is complete I will be a more healthy and pure soul.

Taylor's Diary
November 21, 2000

I now take time out of the day to really experience and savor even the simplest things life has to offer. At this particular moment of the day I am enjoying every second of a James Taylor CD as I watch the most beautiful rays of sunlight dance across my pillow. Today is especially beautiful out; the air is crisp, the setting a beautiful thing for upcoming Thanksgiving and sunlight blanketing every tree and flower. Jeff stopped by before he left for North Carolina. It was just what I needed to brighten my day a little bit more. In all I am feeling peaceful and happy, but my tiredness has gotten the best of me so I must tend to that until next time.

Chapter Five: Thanksgiving

It was a tradition in the family that the extended clan met at Aunt Barbara's in Melbourne for the traditional Thanksgiving dinner. For a number of years I attended these events until my wife released me on waivers, as they say in baseball, although I prefer the phrase, "My wife released me to my future." They were lovely dinners and Barbara was always gracious, but after the divorce I didn't make the trek.

"How was Thanksgiving at Aunt Barbara's," I remember asking Taylor when she came through the front door after her last such dinner. I don't recall how she replied to my question, but later I read in her diary.

Filled with the comfort of chaos. Dysfunction ran abundant both in the car ride up and the actual Thanksgiving dinner. We are a family that puts the "fun" in dysfunction. It was a line Taylor often used and it implied a bit of obliviousness as well. She was actually much more concerned about another matter; she was more concerned about Jeff. *That* conversation I remember.

Jeff the boyfriend. Always Jeff the boyfriend. A seventeen-year-old girl could be obsessed with her boyfriend and I remember how self-conscious Taylor was because of her cancer. Well, I was certainly glad Jeff wasn't Erik, a previous beau. Now there was a loser. "What's up?" I asked her.

"Jeff's acting weird," she replied. "He left me on hold for at least ten minutes and hasn't called me back since. I hung up and am debating whether to call him or not. But to call him would expose my weakness to him, wouldn't it?"

I didn't say anything. I don't think she wanted me to.

I read in her diary her lament: *And my hair is coming out in drastic amounts.* I remember her adding that comment. That was so true. We had been warned about the side effects of the chemo and sure enough, clumps of hair were beginning to fall out of Taylor's scalp. If it was unnerving to her father, I realized, it was terrifying to her. Taylor had a beautiful head of hair, worthy of a cover girl. To lose such a mark of beauty was devastating for a seventeen-year-old girl. She was surprisingly philosophical about it though. I remember reading an entry in her diary:

Maybe losing my hair is absolutely essential for me to reach a higher level or understanding and acceptance in this lesson God is trying to teach me, she wrote. Maybe I must be stripped of external beauty in order to really create inner beauty. I must remember this every time I walk past a mirror.

I think she wrote that to reassure herself. It was a form of acceptance I realized on rereading the passage; a spiritual transformation was beginning.

A week after that diary entry, Taylor surprised me with a totally bald head. "I shaved my head, Dad," I remember her saying, stating the obvious. "I have a beautiful head, don't I?" she added, preening before a hand-held mirror.

I agreed that she had a beautiful head as she mockingly preened in a mirror like a diva. Then she took my hand and playfully rubbed it across her skull and chuckled at my discomfort.

She wrote in her diary: *It's kind of empowering and humbling at the same time. It is definitely a unique experience. I'm just going to make the best of it, that's my decision. Jeff is wonderful as ever…*

So Jeff was out of her doghouse that day, although he would return to it now and then over the year. It was the mercurial feature of a teenage romance, on-again, off-again, on-again. I always thought if Shakespeare's famous teenagers Romeo and Juliet hadn't killed themselves they probably would have split sometime in the non-existent fourth act. I was a bit too cynical when it came to Jeff. He turned out to be a pretty good egg as I learned later from an entry in Taylor's journal.

I can't help but think it's too good to be true. I mean how can an attractive eighteen-year-old guy stay faithful and emotionally committed to a girl who constantly has some distressing situation or another? I don't know if I should let it just happen. I have tried to give him an out on a few separate occasions but he won't even hear of it. Yesterday, I went over to his house and I got a bit emotional about my impending baldness. He made a remark about how I would still be beautiful and a river of tears came flooding out. He knew exactly what to do and say to comfort me. Maybe he came into my life just in time to help me through.

Maybe he did Taylor. And he left shortly thereafter.

Jeff would outlive Taylor, but only by a few months. In the spring of 2002 he was killed in a daylight automobile accident in North Carolina about two weeks after the *60 Minutes* program aired. He never got a chance to live his dream and join the NASCAR circuit.

* * *

The chemotherapy caused Taylor's long brown hair to fall out. First it was a few hairs, then it was a few strands and then it was clump after clump. It was only when she started losing

21

clumps of her hair that she became despondent. Her hair, like so many teenage girls, was such a part of her. It was if her soul was being drained from her.

With the hair loss came a loss of self-confidence, a feeling that how could her boyfriend still love her? It seemed that all throughout her illness Taylor was more concerned about Jeff's love than her own life. Here is a passage from her diary.

Taylor's Diary
December 4, 2000

Today was a simple but pleasant one. Make that until the evening. Jeff was being a real shit and I felt the need to hang up on him. Needless to say I'm hopeless so I called him back. I haven't had my mind on the "cancer" lately. I've just been living my life as any other normal bald girl. It's quite nice. I haven't showed Jeff my head yet, although I think he'll be really good about it. And that's the true test really, to see if it's real. I don't know why I'm dreading it. Maybe I'm afraid he'll see my bald head and be horrified outright or if not, even worse, he'll pretend not to be bothered, but will never look at me the same again. I just wish that I would have some assurance, because that hurt would not heal easily.

Chapter Six: Twilight on the Beach

When she was younger, of middle school age, Taylor and I would sometimes visit the Hutchinson Island beach at the House of Refuge museum which was once a refuge for shipwrecked sailors off the coast of Florida as early as 1825. It's craggy shore with ocean spraying over the rocks gave the House of Refuge Beach a hint of a northern seashore or perhaps an English shoreline worthy of a Bronte sister novel. Twilight was our favorite time and the House of Refuge Beach was Taylor's favorite site on Hutchinson Island to feel inspired to write her poetry. She had written poetry since she was a little girl; I like to think in some ways that she was emulating me, although choosing her own medium of expression in poetry instead of prose. For fathers dream that their daughters carry on the family association with the muse as they would dream of such for their sons. In fact, there were a number of men in town who had hung up "& daughter" signs on their shingles. Still, I thought, if she were to be a writer in the future I would have to steer her away from the poet's poverty toward the middle class muse of non-fiction feature writing. But back then, when she was eleven on a balmy October Florida evening, I sat next to her on the beach as she worked on a poem that she said would be different.

She was writing in a spiral composition book and the poem was her normal style which was sort of Will Rogers' version of a sonnet: "I never met a couplet I didn't like." Rhyme, rhyme, if she kept this up she would probably wind up writing cards for Hallmark.

I admit to 1) not liking poetry and 2) not understanding most of it, but for the most part I got the drift of Taylor's poems. But this one was a bit precocious for a sixth grader. I remember wondering, *Had she channeled Emily Dickinson?* She loved Dickinson, always had; a volume of the *Belle of Amherst's* verse was on a bookshelf in her old bedroom.

Tales of the Sea by Taylor Black (at age 11)

I was laying on the warm white sand,
And all of the sudden I reached for a hand.
It led me into the water so blue.
And I couldn't help but ask, "who are you?"
He never spoke he just kept on walking,
Then told me a tale which was very shocking.
He said to me "as the waves roll upon the mighty shore
We will go knocking on Time's great door."
And then there I was in a time not my own,
With only a ghost and my own flesh and bone.
"I am here to tell you my tale of the sea,
For there's no one left to tell it but me,
I've been needing to tell this tale for so long,
A human's not cargo I know that today,
But I can't help get over my own soul's dismay,
How could I be so keen with a whip,
Oh the lashes I gave on this cross ocean trip."

Taylor seemed to sense that I was a bit startled by her precocity or perhaps her subject matter and she employed a tactic, which her grandmother had taught her very well: change the subject. I remember her switching gears and asking, "The ocean is amazing, Dad, nature is so amazing, dontcha think?"

"Yes, Tale," I admitted. It was always "dontcha think"—not "don't you," but "dontcha."

As if on cue from the Big Director, the curtain went down on that day and a canopy of stars began to glimmer above us.

"How many stars do you think there are, Dad?" she asked, pointing to the sky.

"Billions and billions," I replied.

"I really don't understand the concept of billions," she said.

No, she never did, I remember. Math! She had to spend one summer in summer school for geometry in high school with Mrs. Hubbard, the best calculus teacher in the state. Interesting how good that teacher was, but then calculus teachers are proficient in all areas of math, and I remember Taylor literally running into the house and, in a "Eureka!" moment, proclaiming, "I understand math!" It was amazing what a great teacher could do, and from that point on, after that summer school sojourn with Mrs. Hubbard, Taylor never had a math problem again, that was, until she ran into something called a debit card, the bane of her bank balance. But that evening on the beach the problems with geometry lay in the future and I was left trying to explain to my middle school daughter what billions were all about.

"Imagine every grain on this beach as a star and then you get the idea, Tale."

"Wow!" She could really make me feel as if I had just said something profound.

"The stars we see tonight may not even be there, what we are seeing may really only be light. We are looking backward in time when we look at the sky." I admit to having felt uncommonly wise at that moment. "And those stars we see twinkling may not even be there anymore," I added.

I received another. "Wow!"

Yes, an eleven-year-old child can make a father feel like a genius. How many times have I explained the concept of light from the stars to my high school students and yet Taylor treated me as a new Einstein. She could make fatherhood sublime with a "wow."

* * *

A week later Taylor came home from school and tossed her book bag on the couch. She was upset.

"My teacher says I took my poem from a book, Dad," she fumed.

I asked her what book.

"Well, she didn't know what book. She said my poem was too good for a student to write. She accused me of stealing the poem."

I sat down and wrote a diplomatic letter to Taylor's English teacher. Handing the note to Taylor, I said. "Take this to your teacher tomorrow." Then I gave her a hug.

There were tears in Taylor's eyes, but the tears were not from sadness, but from anger. Taylor didn't cheat. Hell, she had the report cards to prove it. She loved the whole alphabet not just the letter *A* and she had received all four of the first letters of the alphabet in middle school. Later, in a biology class at Indian River Community College, the professor had students "grade themselves" and everyone in the class but Taylor gave themselves an *A*; Taylor gave herself a *C*, and those were the grades that were posted in that class. Twenty-one *A*'s I guess and one lone *C*, Taylor's, and I was never more proud of her for that act of integrity, but I remember telling her not to think about a career in the U.S. Congress.

In sixth grade, Taylor would get through the year in English class but she would never respect her English teacher again, and neither would I.

A few years ago I watched a DVD of the film *Amazing Grace* about William Wilberforce's fight to abolish slavery in Britain and learned the author of one the greatest hymns I had ever sung was a repentant slave ship captain, John Newton, who would go on to become a minister as well as a prolific hymn composer. I wish Taylor could have seen that movie and I sometimes wonder if the spirit of that British slave ship captain visited her that night on the beach.

On December 23, 2009, two days before Taylor's favorite day of the year, I was cleaning up her old bedroom so Courtney could paint over the Tiger tracks Taylor had splashed on her walls when I came across some keepsakes of my late mother's. There was Taylor's poem "Tales of the Sea" among Nana's little treasures, neatly typed by the author. I had lost my copy of the poem some years ago. In the mail that same day my stepdaughter Jenni sent me a note and Taylor's handwritten copy of the same poem. In my program we sometimes say that "coincidences are God's way of working anonymously." Either God or a little angel. At least that's what I believe.

Taylor's Diary
December 11, 2000

I had chemo this weekend. I don't really write in here (the hospital) through chemo because I think of it like this: the

*time before and after the hospital is training for a match &
then in the hospital is being in the ring, so you've just got to
go for the K.O. Anyway, I got back last night but I was
feeling rather poorly. Today I pretty much slept/rested (didn't
stay asleep much) and then Jeff came over. Well, I have a
mountain of work to do tomorrow so I'm gonna sleep.*

While she was taking chemotherapy Taylor was trying to
finish her classes at Indian River Community College. She was
enrolled in dual enrollment and was taking college classes at
the junior college while still in high school. The plan was to let
her finish the fall classes at the college and then transfer her to
"homebound" for her last semester of high school. Her sister
Beth, an art teacher, and I would give Taylor instruction in two
classes as we traveled to Duke University and other hospitals
which would allow Taylor to graduate with her high school
class on time. Still, even though it was difficult to juggle
chemotherapy with college economics, Taylor always seemed
to find time to socialize. But in this diary entry, she waxes
philosophical.

Taylor's Diary
December 18, 2000

*Well, I was in the middle of cleaning my horribly messy
room but I stopped and picked you up (her diary). Why does
it take forever to clean my room and why do I keep
everything? Anyway, this weekend was very interesting. On
Sat. night I went out w/ Jeff and Mike (and Ted) but anyway
it was all very strange, having both Mike and Jeff there. It
was sort of bringing together my past and my present.
Somehow it put me @peace. I was listening to oldies today
when "Ohhh Child" came on. I was knocked down by joy and*

began to cry. As tears were streaming down my face I felt contentment and the greatness of my life. It is only through my obstacles and triumphs that I can feel the penetrating core of life. Today I thought I haven't been writing poetry. I know I still have some feelings that I need to work through, but I don't want to have a breakdown 'til after the holidays. It won't really be too drastic, but I'll have to work out a few minor details. Until later.

Chapter Seven: Lions and Tigers and Bears Oh My!

Maybe Taylor's creativity began years before that during story hour at bedtime.

Taylor was six and Courtney was eight and they shared a bedroom at my house, a complex which I referred to as the "duplexes of the divorced dads with visitation rights." At Pam's house, the girls also shared a bedroom, but their bedroom on Seashell Lane was larger than at my duplex. And at the duplex they shared a trundle bed and every night they were with me, we had story time. The opening story was, invariably, *The Tortoise and the Hare* in which I played the parts of the tortoise, the hare and the hare's girlfriend played by Taylor. It was a nightly ritual. I always said, "And the hare was far, far ahead so he decided to stop and a pretty girl rabbit came by and said...Taylor?"

Taylor stood up on the lower portion of the trundle bed and like some little girl at a beauty pageant said in a vain attempt at a husky voice, "How ya doing big boy?"

"Very good, Taylor" I whispered and she smiled.

"And they started to kiss," Taylor added with a big giggle and began to mimic a number of kissing gestures.

I would always continue with, "The rabbit said, 'oh, my gosh, oh my gosh. I'm in a race. I'm in a race!' And he went zoom, zoom," I said, tickling Taylor's tummy, and she giggled even louder in delight. Courtney laughed as well when I tickled her. "And the turtle just kept crawling and just at the last second as he neared the finish line he stuck his head out of his shell and won the race."

"Yeah!" Taylor clapped would always clap, but one night she asked, "Can we make up a story, Daddy?"

I remember thinking, *Why not?* There wasn't a "bedtime stories rulebook" that I knew of, but I decided to stay with animals just to be on the safe side. I mean it was good enough for Aesop right? I began, "Okay, there once was a kangaroo and an elephant. Courtney?"

"And they lived in the jungle," Courtney added.

Well, so now our story became intercontinental, mixing Australian marsupials with African pachyderms. I decided to let it slide.

"Taylor?" I said.

"And they could fly." Taylor said, raising her hands and flapping them for effect.

"That's dumb. They can't fly," Courtney said.

"Dumbo can," Taylor said, holding her ground. "And my elephant can too. Can't he, Daddy?"

"Kangaroos can't fly, stupid." Courtney persisted.

"They might, right, Daddy?" Taylor said to me.

I was caught between sisters in the DMZ, or the "Daddy, Me! Zone," not a good place for a father to be. Courtney was my logical child with a good imagination and Taylor was my illogical child with a good imagination. She was the youngest and I had been the youngest and there was a soft spot in my heart for her because of her birth order. Only an adult who was the youngest child can really appreciate his youngest child, I always thought. There was some special bond there, but at that moment it didn't help. Both of the girls looked at me to act as a referee on the flying abilities of elephants and kangaroos.

Solomon had it easy with that baby. Just split the difference. Hey, Solomon, try settling a dispute among your five hundred daughters; they would have driven your right out of the Old Testament.

And I might have thought, *What would Jesus do,* but in my mind my mother's visage lit up my thought: Wisdom from Nana.

"How about tomorrow night we go to McDonald's for dinner?" I said, ducking the issue like a seasoned politician.

Taylor looked at me like a pint-sized prosecutor. "You changed the subject, Daddy. That's what Nana does." Taylor, of course, would use Nana's dictum on me when in middle school.

"I love Nana," Taylor said, and she was obviously not thinking about flying animals but rather about summer at her grandmother's. She reached over and hugged Courtney and gave her a goodnight kiss. "I love you, Courtney," she said.

And at the moment in my mind a kangaroo and elephant were dancing across the sky.

Taylor's Diary
December 20, 2000

Praise the Lord! I am finished with exams. I feel as if a 500 lb. block was lifted from my shoulders. Well, it is only 5 days 'till Christmas. It's funny, but this year I'm really into the spirit, which I love. It's almost like you need to have a drastic measure to truly appreciate the simple magical things. Although I did a horribly stupid thing today by trying to brave the holiday crowds. It was a last minute part of Jeff's present. Of course, I didn't find anything and it wiped me out. I slept for 3 hours. All that for a guy that hasn't even called me back yet. Oh well, I suppose I will talk w/him tomorrow. Katie came over yesterday when I was just lying down and I was extremely curt with her. But I decided I'm not gonna feel bad because she has been really shitty during this whole thing and I'm extremely hurt by it. Well, what do I have to complain about? Life is beautiful! It really is. Everyone needs to remember that at least once every day because it is so short and so precious and to take it for granted is the biggest sin any soul can commit.

Taylor's Diary
December 21, 2000

Mother, I know at times you try,
But sometimes not enough,
And even when I cry
I only get rebuffed.

Taylor's Diary
December 23, 2000

Well, the countdown continues to Christmas. Jeff got me the most beautiful diamond heart necklace. I love it. I was just lying down w/him last night. Just lying there, nothing else, and it felt so incredibly amazing like I belonged with him. It was like going home. Does that mean that I'm in love w/him or he's the one? But the thing is that I don't get tired of him, I could have him around for a long time. Although some things don't fit perfectly, that's natural but he's really something else. Anyway, enough about that. Can you believe tomorrow's Christmas Eve. Oh, I just absolutely love it. It is perhaps the best time of year.

P.S. I think the writing ability has left me or perhaps I never had it. All my poems are garbage!

I always thought Taylor could be too hard on herself at times. I have written professionally for years, but I doubt if my prose would be up to snuff it cancer was eating at my brain. Still, she might have moments of self-doubt, but she couldn't give up her couplet rhymes, although her Christmas entry said otherwise.

Taylor's Diary
December 25, 2000

Sometimes I feel like I am a totally unoriginal average person w/nothing to offer the world, I know, very enlightening realization on this holiday. I need to start being an active person, you know, & truly metamorphose. Right not it's just all clutter and lard and I really need to work on that. Another thing: why can't I write anymore?

Chapter Eight: Right Field Is Where the Dandelions Grow

After Taylor's brain surgery at Martin Memorial Hospital in Stuart, she resumed her night classes at Indian River Community College. I enjoyed driving her to class as it gave us some time to be alone together. Those evenings became very special to both of us. We talked and Taylor often repeated how she appreciated every minute of every day, especially the sunsets.

"I really feel alive, Dad," Taylor said one evening. She added with a smile. "I was just remembering when you hit me with a softball."

"Nuts," I said. "I thought maybe they cut *that* painful memory out in the brain surgery."

She laughed, but at the time I beaned her, the incident didn't seem so funny. It was downright embarrassing.

Taylor was eight and the smallest softball player on the Langford Park Red Sox of a beginner's league on which her father was the assistant coach. Mike Jordan was the head coach and he was a Red Sox fan so the team was named for the Beantown Boys. I would have taken the Phillies as our team name, but assistants didn't get to choose. So Mike's girls, great athletes, and my daughters, a bit deficient in athletic acumen, played on the team with Courtney relegated to left field and Taylor to right. Balls were seldom hit to the outfield at this age and a grounder to third was nearly always a single as none of the girls could throw across the diamond. Normally, the first girl up made it to first base and from then on most of the outs were recorded with force outs at second.

And the fathers pitched because the young girls lacked the control to get a ball consistently over the plate. In the case of Taylor, that really didn't matter, for she had managed to hit the ball only a few times all season and those were foul balls. In fact she had struck out nearly every time, save for a walk once or twice I believe. Taylor really didn't care about softball; she was our team's Lucy Van Pelt. When on defense, she sat in right field and picked dandelions. Sometimes she danced after a butterfly like some pint-sized Isadora Duncan frolicking on a crab grass stage. Right field was her own little world and it was amusing for an adult to watch Taylor show such indifference to a game in progress. Something, however, was at progress in Taylor's mind. *But why not ignore the game?* I thought. There was only one left-handed batter who might possibly have hit the ball to right field and she was on our team. Taylor may have been unconcerned about the game but she wanted to be part of the team because Katie and Karly, her best friends, were on the squad. Karly was a so-so softballer but Katie was a star, a regular distaff version of Pete Rose, although Katie would never get caught betting on the games in our league.

So one night, when Mike Jordan was away on a business trip, I was elevated to the exalted position of head coach with the added responsibility of "steady pitcher." I penciled in the lineup. Taylor was batting last, of course.

I was having control problems as bad as Tim Robbins in *Bull Durham* and in the bottom of the second my youngest daughter arrived at the plate, the aluminum bat on her tiny shoulder. I had already nearly beaned two girls—thankfully we didn't have a mascot for me to bean—but those tykes had the common sense and good coordination to move before the ball hit them. And now I was about to pitch to the pomegranate of my eye and I reared back and tossed the sphere underhand toward the plate but the ball's trajectory was errant and I yelled, "Move, Taylor."

Taylor chose that moment to try out for team statue. The ball plunked off her left shoulder. She did not drop her bat, she stayed in position. She was indeed a statue, except statues don't cry.

"Child abuse!" a smart aleck father yelled from the stands.

Thanks pal, I really needed that, I remember thinking. I knew the guy and I wanted to race into the stands and give him a knuckle sandwich, but hey I was supposed to be a grown-up wasn't I? Right. Men are never grownups. We are still ten-year-old boys inside when we step on a baseball diamond. But my guilt in plunking my daughter grew with every nanosecond.

"Take your base, honey," the umpire told Taylor, but she stood as still as Michelangelo's marble, the tears rolling down her face, the disbelief filling her eyes. My father hit me with the ball, her contorted face seemed to proclaim. My own daddy! Slowly, with the help of some unseen Aphrodite of athletics, the statue pulled a Galatea and became ambulatory and began a slow walk to first base, rubbing her left shoulder with her right arm. I felt awful. Oh, it's not that I hadn't spanked her before. She made the term "terrible twos" an extension of alliteration as in Taylor's terrible tantrums at two and her bottom had been warmed on more than one occasion during that trying annum as my palm had nearly hit heating pad status, but to hit her with a ball? Only a cad, a cur or some other type of wretch would hit his daughter with a softball.

Taylor learned a thing about adults that day as well; they lie. Softballs are not soft, they are hard, at least when they hit you. A Nerf Ball? That's soft. A beanbag? That's soft. A softball isn't soft.

I called time and walked penitently to first base. I took a deep breath and looked at my bewildered little girl. "Are you okay, Tale?" I asked.

She nodded. Thank heavens the tears had stopped. It always amazed me that there weren't more women plumbers in the world, for a girl could turn a faucet of tears on and off so easily. I hugged her. Normally it was Taylor who initiated the hugs, Taylor who seemed to need the hugs, this time, I needed the hugs.

The Red Sox lost once again, 23-17. We didn't have a closer.

Chapter Nine: A Father's Worst Fear

On September 22, 2000, my ex-wife Pam took Taylor to the emergency room after she fainted in a shower at Pam's house. Her mother's intuition kicked in and I was glad of it for what was about to begin. The following day, Taylor began a diary of her experiences.

I realized, when I reread her first entry from that life-altering night when the brain tumor was discovered, that Taylor culled her diaries and used portions of her journals when she delivered a speech at the Swan Hotel in Disneyworld at the American Cancer Society Convention two days before the terrorist attack on the United States of America.

On the afternoon of the 23rd, Taylor returned to my house and told me what had happened. Our world, as we had known it, had suddenly changed. She would later write that the light seemed to go out of my eyes at the moment when she told me she had a brain tumor. I don't recall that. I recall being stunned, as if someone had sucker-punched me in the stomach. There are so many moments that I wish I was able to relive, because the shock of the moment was so devastating it seemed to wipe out some of the images, like photographic film being exposed to a blinding light. I remember saying to Taylor, "You can beat this," with a voice that tried for authority, but I'm sure rang hollow with doubt and fear. *She* was certainly frightened. I was terrified. Was the brain tumor benign or malignant? That was the question. The tumor in her head was the size of a peach. I remember trying to shake the image of a peach out of my mind. Why couldn't it have been the size of a cherry? Or a pea? Maybe then I wouldn't have been so terrified. A peach seemed so big to me. A few days later, a day before Taylor's scheduled surgery, Taylor wrote in her journal.

The past few days have been a whirlwind. It's like a haze has come over me. Everyone is sending cards and calling. They look at me as if they have just run over my puppy. It is a look that reaffirms the magnitude of what is happening. I feel like I need to wake up from a nightmare.

I remember her saying something like that to me at the time and "I know" was all I could reply. But I didn't *know* squat. I realized she just wanted me to listen to her vent about the things she had no control over. My daughters had taught me the lesson of listening to women which is often so difficult for a man; a man wants to fix it, right then and there. And sometimes there is no fix or the woman is working out her own solution to a problem by talking about it. That was what Taylor was doing at that moment.

I guess you could say this is the antithesis of Christmas, Taylor wrote. *Besides the whole tumor thing, this would be a pleasant time. Missing school and seeing everyone. Doctors and tests, doctors and tests. They are not even sure what kind of tumor it is. This seems so unreal. Until last week, I never spent the night in a hospital and now I'm going in for brain surgery. Maybe after I do this then it will all turn out to be no big deal and everyone will feel stupid for getting crazy over nothing.*

She went on to write about her beautiful long hair; she wanted to keep her hair. What seventeen-year-old girl wanted to lose her hair? The next day after that journal entry she was scheduled for eight hours of brain surgery and I remember kissing her cheek and taking my leave to allow her to gather things for her hospital stay.

Her sisters were throwing a pre-brain surgery pizza party in her hospital room when I arrived a bit later that evening. Taylor had a brave little smile as the twins teased her about a number of things not related to her impending surgery. I marveled at how close sisters were, unlike my brothers and I, who were never really tight. There was something about sisters I realized in that moment, for the sisters of this sibling sorority had drawn a protective curtain around their youngest member and were trying to give her strength for her upcoming ordeal. I realize women are superior to men in that regard: caring for others. It was so obvious in that hospital room that night, when all my daughters, both step and biological were all there together, drawing strength from each other with our own family version of *Steel Magnolias.* Oh, the girls welcomed me, all of them, but my presence certainly wasn't necessary, and after a few minutes I walked over to Taylor and gave her another kiss on the cheek. She smiled again, looked straight into my eyes as if surveying my soul, and grabbed my hand and gave it a squeeze as if to reassure *me* that everything was going to be okay. Sometimes things are said through the silence of a look and this was one of those times.

But it was only beginning. The next fourteen months would be the greatest challenge of all our lives as Taylor would document in her journal.

Chapter Ten: Dad Starts a Journal

I agreed to keep a journal through her ordeal as a companion to Taylor's diary. From brain surgery to recovery, that sort of thing, journals that would someday become something of an "Anne Frank and Dad" of cancer, something that might help other people face the disease, to show how *we* coped, how *we* overcame, how *we* triumphed, because, of course, *we* were special, *we* were the chosen ones, the ones who would beat cancer like cyclist Lance Armstrong. After all, things didn't happen to *us*, they happened to that vague, nebulous group of "other people" but now, suddenly, they had happened to *us*, but *we* of course "were special." My feelings weren't unique, it is something most people feel: being special. Bad things happen to others, not to us, and there I was, keeping my journal for September 29, 2000.

"My daughter Taylor entered Martin Memorial last night. Brain surgery was scheduled for today at 7 a.m. and the operation should last until the early afternoon. Brain surgery! Lord, in heaven, why Taylor?

"The waiting room is filled with Vaughn Monroe memorabilia: the Big Band leader's RCA jacket, two 78 RPMS and a trumpet, a photo and an oil painting given by his family after he died in the hospital in 1973. None of the younger family members give a fig about Vaughn Monroe or even have a clue who he was. 'That paths of glory lead but to the grave,' Thomas Gray once wrote. That epigram certainly applied to Big Band leaders. I might add, that one generation's 'star' doesn't necessarily twinkle in the next.

"Family: the room is populated by my ex-in-laws and my stepchildren. Grandma Virginia, sister-in-law Barb and my

45

brother-in-law Ronnie. Cousin Lisa, Courtney. My stepdaughter Tracey and twin stepdaughters, Jenni and Beth. Taylor's brothers: Chad and Todd. Seven children, a large Catholic family.

"But I need sunglasses for the glares from my ex-wife Pam. And perhaps even a crucifix or some garlic. Even though we have been divorced thirteen years her hatred for me is palpable, but I am too concerned about Taylor to engage in our own version of *Family Feud*. It is amazing to think that this surly faced woman is a person I once adored and with whom I created two lovely daughters, the youngest of whom is under the surgeon's scalpel at that moment. How did loving turn to loathing? That's a story for another day, I think. I do something nearly impossible for me when I see her: I keep my mouth shut.

"The family chit-chats about nothing, as if the sounds of banality can ease the fear and tension in the room. I bring history essays to grade; there is comfort in correcting grammar, as grammar can be corrected. But can Taylor be corrected? Cousin Lisa, a high school science teacher (who will later become an FBI agent) has a stack of lab reports to mark. Other family members nervously leaf through the out-of-date magazines that dot the waiting room coffee tables and end tables. No one speaks of the operation as if we speak of it we will jinx the surgery. We are a family that avoids discussing difficult subjects like alcoholism or substance abuse as if by not talking about our problems they will magically go away, like the end credits on a movie. But unfortunately, there is always a sequel around the corner.

"The head nurse in the operating room comes out after a few hours and speaks to us. Her son is one of my students. It is one of the blessings of a small town like Stuart: the interconnections among the residents. She tells us everything is going along okay and they are "debulking" the tumor. But it is not "encapsulated," a condition we had hoped for as that would indicate the tumor hadn't spread. An "encapsulated" tumor would allow the surgeon to go in, cut it out, and that would be the end of it all with a 'lived happily ever after.' But there is no Fairy Godmother in this scenario, no turning this pumpkin into a royal carriage"

* * *

For Taylor there would be no glass slipper, no "happily ever after," for the tumor was malignant and we would be given three different diagnoses over the ensuing days which, I must admit, tested my faith in the medical system. How can one feel confident with a diagnosis de jour? I believe even Job might not have enough patience for this.

Courtney, Taylor's closest sibling, would be the most affected, both short term and long term. As Taylor was led to ICU for recovery, Courtney walked beside me down the hospital corridor to the exit and did something she hadn't done in years; she took my hand and looked at me with moist eyes as if asking me for reassurance but silently realizing I had none to offer. I felt like such a failure as a father. All I could offer Courtney were my tears.

Sometimes Taylor comes to me in my present thoughts and tells me, *You weren't a failure as a father, Pops. You have to know that, Pops. It was out of your control.*

I reply that I know, but I still felt that way.

And her voice invariably reminds me, *Feelings pass, Pops. Just like people do.*

Chapter Eleven: Cinderella's Castle

Taylor was in ICU post brain tumor operation. Tubes were up her nose. She was in the arms of Morpheus, the mythical god of sleep. She appeared so peaceful. Tranquility Base, my eaglet has landed, I remember thinking.

I just sat there beside her in the ICU after her first brain surgery and held her hand. I thought, *I'm a good father. I protect my girls. Once again I felt like a failure. This was all so wrong. Hell, I smoked for 30 years. I should have the cancer, like my father who died of lung cancer in 1974 because he couldn't kick the cigarette habit. Shit! Not Taylor! Why God?? Why Taylor??* It is a question without an answer, at least in this lifetime, but it is on the top of my list in case St. Peter meets me with, "Do you have any questions?" Of course I might wind up in the "other place."

Get back to the story, Pops, Taylor says in my mind. *You're digressing.* She was always catching me when I digressed in a story.

Flowers were everywhere in the ICU. What is it with flowers? We give them to the sick, we give them to brides, we give them to the dead and we give them to our mothers. There is a language of flowers, a vernacular known to females and the FTD Mercury guy, and like most men I am illiterate. Taylor had a rainbow of colors in the intensive care unit. Remember "Rainbow Bright," Taylor? I asked my sedated daughter.

As if on cue Taylor wakes up and smiled at me. I squeezed her hand. She squeezed back. The squeeze was surprisingly strong.

In my mind it is 1974. My sixty two-year-old father was on his death bed at Bryn Mawr Hospital. His cancer metastasized and caused a blood clot and a resultant stroke that impaired his speech. Then the pneumonia infiltrated his lungs. He could only squeeze my hand to communicate as the stroke had left him speechless, a man who was the international president of a labor union, who was accustomed to addressing a couple thousand union members in convention hall. Dad was in *Who's Who in America* but he couldn't even speak to me and there was so much left unsaid between us, so much forgiveness that needed to be shared and was shared, I suppose, in the gentle squeezing of hands between a father and a son. In my mind as I sat in the ICU I saw my father's palsied face, but it changed into Taylor's. My father, my daughter; I shivered. I couldn't stay long: There were other family members waiting and we could only have two people in at a time in ICU. And I wanted to be alone with her.

I asked God to help Taylor that night and I tried not to be angry with Him. What was the name of that play? *Your Arms Too Short to Box with God*? But that didn't mean I didn't want to throw a punch at old Yahweh.

People all over Martin County began praying for Taylor. The second grade at St. Joseph's. Catholics. Jews. Fundamentalist Protestants. My brother the Quaker started prayers at the Friends meeting in Brooklyn. I called Jim, my Mormon friend, in Utah. Taylor was put on the Mormon prayer list. I figured it couldn't hurt to be ecumenical. Everyone was praying for Taylor. Only seventeen. Why Taylor, God? Why us?

I remember sitting there in the ICU and thinking of Cinderella's Castle at Disneyworld. The girls liked that mythological castle when they were young. Every little girl's dream programmed by the silly fantasy that Prince Charming would make everything right, that a man would save the woman every time. Hallmark hogwash Disney denial, I would diagnosis it. When Taylor was little and posing with Courtney in front of Cinderella's Castle, she once asked me, "In the movies why doesn't the girl ever save the boy, Daddy?" I answered in real life the girls often save the boys, Taylor, and sometimes the boys don't even know it.

On my wall in my den as I write this sentence is the poster of Taylor at 5 and Courtney at 7 standing at Disneyworld with Cindy's Castle in the background. It is a picture I took that came out so well I had it blown up into a poster and laminated so that it wouldn't fade over the years as my memories have. In that poster, the girls are pre-Piaget age of reason rug rats who believed in Santa Claus—or Sandy Claws as Taylor used to call him. They also believed in the Easter Bunny and the Valentine Bird, an invention of their maternal grandfather, who created the avian of amour as an excuse to indulge his granddaughters with more candy and himself with a half-gallon of vodka.

But back in ICU...I guess my mind wandered off to thoughts of Disneyworld and Cinderella's Castle that night because the fantasy of the Magic Kingdom was preferable to the reality of a daughter in an ICU. I knew that we were certainly going to need a touch of magic in the coming days and I wished Tinker Bell would show up and sprinkle some fairy dust so Taylor could fly away to Never Never Land, or that we would wake up and all of this would be merely a bad dream.

* * *

For Taylor Y2K turned out to be as bad as many had predicted, although her computer didn't crash in 2000, but having a brain tumor operation can kind of besmirch even the best of years and although she had a boyfriend she also had chemotherapy. Still everyone was hopeful as 2001 began, especially Taylor.

Taylor's Diary
January 2, 2001

Well, so begins a new year. Maybe this one will be better than the last. I can't help but wonder what twists and turns life has in store for me this year, but I know I can handle whatever comes my way. I went to the doctor's today. All my counts are good which is always good news, but Dr. McArthur says he wanted me to go to Duke w/in the next week & when I go I have to stay for 7-10 days. What a nice B-day present that would be huh? Well, I suppose there are far worse things. I can't get all worked up about it. After all it's only as bad as you make it out to be. At times it is extremely difficult to not wallow in self-pity, but in those moments you must rise above and take heed of the lesson you are receiving. Because after all isn't that what great tragedies and triumphs really are: lessons to be learned? So, I suppose for now I'll keep my eyes open and await my teaching.

Taylor's Diary
January 8, 2001

Today was the most beautiful day of the year thus far. I went to the beach and walked to the inlet. The sun was shining brilliantly on the ocean, which was a thousand different shades of blue and green. It was definitely one of God's most spectacular creations. I have to go to Duke soon for the stem cell harvesting (something I'm not @ all looking forward to). Apparently I have to get an MRI beforehand. In all everything's been good lately except I have had two little upsetting moments. They passed and I picked myself up. I am confident that I will beat this. It only wins if you let it win. Otis's mom has been doing Gin-sen Git-su (sp?) sessions w/me. It is method of holistic healing that deals with energy flow in your body. It is very soothing and I have a feeling that it will have positive effects. I haven't seen much of anyone lately. Everybody's in boyfriend mode. Hopefully, I'll hang out w/them soon. Karly and Gia went to Orlando w/o me. I have a feeling they want to move in together, just the two of them. Whatever, life is so short there is no use in letting things like that get to you. You just gotta let things go. I think I'll start doing meditation everyday @ the beach. I think that would be a calming experience. I had the most awful dream about Jeff last night that seemed so real and after I woke up I was uneasy for a couple hours. I hope nothing happened to him today. I'm still waiting to talk to him.

Taylor's Diary
January 11, 2001

Well, today is my 18th birthday and it was not much out of the ordinary. Looking back on this past year my life was very different and promises never to be the same. Well, it is always said that "change is constant." I believe that as long as you embrace the change and allow the twists and turns to teach something there will never be something that you cannot conquer. I know that this whole experience will alter my life forever.

I only hope that I will be able to retain the day to day enrichment I have derived from the whole situation. So, in all, my birthday was a good one. After dinner @ the Olive Garden I went out with Jeff (Mike was there). There are some people you wish would never walk out of your life, but once they have it is impossible for them to make a smooth entry back in. I miss knowing Mike. He is truly a good person.

P.S. I go up to Duke next Thurs. but I have to get a catheter installed in the other side of my chest and I only have to stay up there until the following Wednesday. Then, I think after it's off to Gainesville for radiation.

That was the plan on Taylor's 18th birthday, but the tumor had other plans. The chemotherapy hadn't worked and as a result, the tumor began to grow once more. Taylor would go to Duke, not for a stem cell harvest, but for a second brain tumor operation.

Taylor's Diary
January 23, 2001

Sorry I didn't write before but I had just gotten out of surgery and I had an IV sticking in my arm that made it quite impossible for me to write. So, where should I begin? Well, brain surgery (at Duke) was a surreal experience all together. First, they put me under and then they woke me up. One of the doctors was talking to me for what seemed like an hour, asking me to do various things such as move my arm, tap my hand and other basic motor skills. I was coherent during the operation and then they put me back under and I woke up in intensive care.

So now I'm out of intensive care and out of the hospital waiting in a hotel room @ the University Inn. Tomorrow we are going to have a consultation with Dr. Friedman. We got the pathology back today and Henry Friedman is apparently working out an aggressive game plan. As far as my knowledge of the situation goes they weren't able to extract all of the tumor because that would have damaged vital tissue. So, now I'm pretty much in limbo. My mom mentioned something about doing some of the treatment up here. If anything I think that would be detrimental to my health because I would be out of my element and away from all the systems of support since its mind over matter in a situation like this, every little bit counts. I just need to focus. I know I can beat this. I know I can. It's just gonna be a bitch you know. But every day is one more under the belt. I just need to remember that every night before I go to bed. I'm trying to let this flow through me, but it seems there is something blocking me. For now I can just breathe. Breathe.

The pathology of the tumor was that it was cerebral neuroblastoma with p-net tendencies. The protocol (the method and order of treatment) was: Stem cell harvest one week. Radiation at Shands Hospital at the University of Florida (where sister Courtney was going to school) for 6 weeks and then back to Duke to see where we would go. Eventually the plan would be to put Taylor in the isolation ward for a month or two. But the best laid plans of mice, and men and physicians....

Chapter Twelve: Country Mice

Looking over her journal entry for Taylor's 18th birthday, I began to think of a trip I made with her and Courtney ten years before.

When Taylor was eight and Courtney ten we visited my Brooklyn brother Michael and his wife, Aunt Nancy, using their Lincoln Road limestone as headquarters for a visit to New York City. It was the first time on the subway for my daughters, although they had ridden the train from my mother's house in Wayne into Philadelphia when visiting there. But a New York subway is, shall we say, a bit more challenging than the Paoli Local and my daughters had the fawns-in-the-headlight appearance as we boarded the subway at Prospect Park. The fearsome New Yorkers we envisioned turned out to be rather nice, if somewhat aloof, taking refuge behind a newsprint wall of the "Times" and the "Daily News."

Taylor lost her deer-look quicker than Courtney, not surprisingly. When I would drop them off at the movies, Courtney made Taylor buy the tickets because Taylor was more at ease with strangers, like some pint-sized Blanch Du Bois in *A Streetcar Named Desire*, I thought, although Taylor wasn't a few ants short of a picnic like Tennessee Williams's tragic heroine.

We changed trains like veterans and finally exited at the World Trade Center because the girls wanted to see the city from atop the tallest structures in Manhattan. When I was a boy I had visited the Empire State Building but alas, Meg Ryan never came to my rescue on the observation deck, but then my dad wasn't Tom Hanks either. Of course by 1991,

King Kong had already carried Jessica Lange to the top of the towers, snubbing the once haughty Empire State Building, and the girls had seen that movie and were curious about the towers. That was my fault I guess, for not showing them the Depression Era Fay Wray version of "King Kong" from the 1930s, when Kong climbed what was then derisively called "The Empty State Building."

The World Trade Center building we were on, and I can't remember if it was the North or South tower, seemed to sway ever so slightly, but the girls were excited by the vista. One could literally see for miles and miles. It is still hard for me to fathom that the Towers are gone now.

After the World Trade Center, the three of us were off to the Battery and a boat ride to Miss Liberty. I remember giving the girls a short lecture on Ellis Island as we ferried across the river. I even talked to them about how family names were changed because of the difficulty in communication. A history teacher is, after all, always on call, even in the summer. One never knows when the history teacher will be called upon to cite some obscure fact!

Liberty Island was very crowded. "Stay together and don't wander off," I ordered.

Foolish father. Liberty Island was the largest right field in the world to Taylor. Where were the dandelions? Where were the butterflies? Let us have a dance to summer, to life!

I turned around and Taylor was missing. She had danced off to somewhere.

I asked Courtney where Taylor was.

Courtney was as startled as I, but not totally surprised. Courtney knew her little sister better than anyone, and she knew Taylor had a habit of wandering off on her own. Her brother Chad had had the same wanderlust, often walking away from kindergarten to go home and grab his fishing pole and head for the creek. There were seven kids in the blended family after all, and sometimes we came up short in the head count. Try running a household with seven kids. It ain't easy, but it is always interesting. But that day on Liberty Island I only had two of the rascals and I should have had a tighter rein.

I searched for the panic button and found it. "We've got to find her!" I shouted. I thought, *she couldn't have gone ahead to the pedestal could she?* Where the @#@# was she!

"Relax, Dad," Courtney said evenly, trying to calm her stressed out father. "She'll turn up. She always does."

Not for thirty minutes she didn't. I remember thinking I would need Grecian Formula after this outing. I would be a strawberry blond no more. We scoured the island and then Courtney spotted Taylor, sitting on a bench, crying. I ran over to her and hugged her.

"You left me!" she wailed.

"No we didn't, Tale," Courtney intervened. "You walked off again."

"Courtney," I said, trying to regain parental decorum. "Hold Taylor's hand. We are going to climb the @#@# steps to the statue to visit the @#@# crown."

My children looked startled by my choice of words. But then Taylor perked up as if she smelled adventure, exploration. The faucet which was on her face turned off. No more tears.

The climb to the crown was laborious but it wasn't exhausting as it took a minute for every step upward or so it seemed. Talk about taking one small step for man. An endless chain of people were climbing to Lady Liberty's crown as if all of the "tired, and poor and huddled masses" were yearning to breathe fresh air in Liberty's tiara and had taken that particular day to show up. We were certainly not going to stop. Did Sir Edmund Hillary quit on Mount Everest? The family that climbed together stayed together.

At the summit we spent perhaps two minutes looking out of Liberty's crown at the port of New York in the distance. The view was worth the hike to the top, and one more historical-site was checked off our must-see list, joining Sagamore Hill, Teddy Roosevelt's Oyster Bay home, which we had visited only the day before. My daughters were pleased we climbed to the crown; it would be something to talk about during show and tell when school resumed in August.

On the subway back to Brooklyn, during rush hour, two kind New Yorkers gave up their seats for my daughters and everything was going well until we crossed the river into Brooklyn and the train stopped.

"Everyone out!" a conducted shouted.

"Bomb scare," someone whispered.

Transit police entered the car and ushered the passengers out. Taylor and Courtney looked startled, looking to me for a sign of what to do.

Heck if I knew, it was my first bomb scare too. I grabbed each girl by a hand and exited the subway train and followed the other passengers up the stairs to the street level. I decided to call my brother. Bring in the cavalry to pick us up, I thought. He would arrive on his steed, albeit a VW bug, but a metaphorical steed nonetheless. I found a pay phone and dialed a number. My professor brother answered. Ah, the safety, support and the bosom of my family. Surely Mike would drive out to rescue us! I explained our plight and I remember his words of comfort all of these years later.

"There should be a bus coming to that corner within ten minutes."

So much for the rescue. That was New York after all, and brother Mike might have lost his cherished parking space on his street. What is a bomb scare in comparison to a lost parking spot? So we caught the bus and I simmered inside. I had two little girls and we've just had a bomb scare. We are country mice! We aren't city mice. We are country mice!

I guess Taylor sensed my tenseness for she took that moment to snuggle up to me on the bus. "I love you, Daddy," she said and gave me her little hand to squeeze. Courtney gave me a hug as well.

I decided not to get angry with my brother. What good would it do? We weren't accustomed to sirens at 3 a.m. We left New York the following morning and the girls never returned during their childhood.

A while ago at a family reunion I told this story to my brother Michael's son Wade. He laughed and assured me that he wouldn't have given up his parking spot either. Family was one thing, Wade said, but a parking spot in New York City was hard to come by. But then, my nephew is a city mouse.

Taylor's Diary
January 24, 2001

Well, as I write to you now I am on an airplane heading back to Stuart (they told us that if we didn't take tonight's flight we'd be stuck in Raleigh til Sat.) and as you can imagine that was just not happening. So after quite a frantic bit of running around we were able to make the flight. I feel so bad for my dad though, his whole purpose in coming was to meet w/Friedman and he didn't even get a chance to do that (thanks to the red-head: Taylor's mom). So we had consultation w/Friedman who said that we could go home for a few days (maybe a week if I'm real lucky). But after that I have to come back up for stem cell harvest and then straight to Shands for radiation. The ball park time frame we're looking @ here is about 6 more months which is doable I suppose. Oh yeah, by the way Georgia, Dr. Friedman's intern, also happens to be the star basketball player for the Duke Women's team, so she had a film crew following her around and they got my little bald-headed consultation on camera, which I think bothered Court more than it bothered me, although she was the only one looking beautiful. That's okay because I've been ugly for about 6 months now, a fact that I'm just gonna have to deal w/I expect. In all, my trip to North Carolina was (as usual) one of anticipation upon returning home. And considering that I don't have a lot more time left @ home I need to savor every minute of it. Right now I am filled w/anxiety about everything. I wonder if Jeff and I will be able to make it through all the time apart. What if he gets used to not having a girlfriend around. I mean really he is a very sexy 18 yr. old guy who has girls throwing themselves @ him even now with me around. Is it really fair for me to ask him to put his senior year on hold just because his girlfriend has cancer? I tell myself that whatever happens, happens, but I am so into him now that I would be devastated to lose him. And what if he just stays w/me so as not to hurt me. I mean really what guy is gonna want to hurt a girl in my situation. I suppose I shouldn't even begin to think about that because that will surely drive me mad. Right now, and for a while, all my energy needs to be focused on kicking some major ass (something I'm sure I can do) and for the time being I need to use every available asset and Jeff is definitely one of them. Really, he came into my life right before all of this happened and he hasn't bailed yet. I think that before God puts you in a trying situation like this he gives you all the necessary tools to prevail. You just have to recognize what is needed to fix what. Among my many assets is my amazing family. I was definitely fated that I would have this network of people so incredibly filled with love and hope. If they aren't a major advantage I don't know what is. And although I may have the rarest of the rarest of the rare, I'm twelve steps ahead of everyone w/the people I've got.

Looking out for Taylor was a collective effort. One of the things which we knew was that a patient needs an advocate when she is in the hospital. Pam and I took turns on the Duke trips, with sisters Courtney, Tracey, Jennifer and Beth all taking a turn. Aunt Barbara and grandmother Virginia were indispensable as well. Courtney would become the primary caregiver in early 2001, forgoing a semester at the University of Florida to care for Taylor and get her to her radiation treatments at Shands Hospital.

Chapter Thirteen: It's a Wonderful Life

Scanning the video shelves at the Blake Library for a DVD to take home, I chanced upon a copy of *It's a Wonderful Life*; there were Jimmy Stewart and Donna Reed on the plastic case. *Bedford Falls*, I thought wistfully, and I was suddenly back in my own fantasy world of the past at tinsel time. We would watch the movie one last time at the last Christmas before she died, but I was thinking of an earlier time in her life, B.C., before cancer.

Taylor was fourteen and we were sitting in our living room about to watch a video:

It's a Wonderful Life with Jimmy and Donna. It was one of our Christmas Rituals, along with Taylor's trimming of the small artificial tree. I finally threw that artificial tree away last year as Courtney and I never brought it out in all the Christmas's since Taylor's last. When she left us, it was as if Santa Claus, Rudolph, Elves, the holiday cards, the notes, the presents beneath the artificial tree and the whole tinsel works went with her when she passed on; but when she was fourteen, in the words of Frank Sinatra, it was a very good year.

Taylor had microwaved the popcorn and was liberally seasoning the mix with butter spray and indeed, the few holiday decorations around the house are due to Taylor. She had her mother's "ho ho" Christmas spirit. I pushed the play button and the movie began once again.

"Do you think Clarence will earn his wings, Tale?" I asked her. Yes, it was a stupid question to ask of a child who had seen the movie a dozen times, but it was our ritual icebreaker for the movie. She normally answered with "I hope so," but that time she responded with, "Do you think there really are angels, Dad?"

Her reply caught me up short. I hesitated and then answered. "Seems to me there must be." In my mind I thought, *You're my angel.* I wish now that I had said that to her, but I had no idea how true that thought would become.

Taylor agreed with me about angels and then asked, "Have you ever wondered what life would be like if *you* hadn't been born, Dad?"

I remember telling her, "I guess you wouldn't be here then either."

Her perplexed face told me that was something she hadn't considered. Her existence was predicated on my own. "Wow!" she finally said. "I didn't think of that."

"Boo!" I hissed at the screen, for Mr. Potter has made his first appearance. Long before there was the Grinch, there was Mr. Potter. Lionel Barrymore, Drew Barrymore's ancestor, made a great villain.

"Do you think Mr. Potter is that way because he can't walk and he takes it out on everyone else?" Taylor asked me.

I had never thought of *that* before. I had merely thought of Potter as a Christmas villain. A person didn't need to analyze with a Frank Capra film, one only needed to "feel." "Maybe," I replied, wondering where she was going with the thought. Then she added, like the knee-jerk liberal that she was,

"That's wrong. He shouldn't take his pain out on others."

"You're right." I agreed.

"I wouldn't do that if something happened to me."

"No I don't think you would, Taylor. Not you."

Courtney joined us in the living room and rolled her eyes at the television screen. She was sixteen and a tad more cynical than either Taylor or I.

"Geez, guys, that dumb movie again."

"It's Christmas, Courtney," Taylor said.

"You two are sentimental saps," Courtney said, but it was a seasonal criticism with a pinch of love. And after a few minutes even the jaded Courtney was into empathy for George Bailey's plight.

"Potter is a real creep isn't he?" Courtney said. "Has Uncle Billy lost the money yet?"

I remember deciding to try for a teaching parallel, "Have I told you girls about the story of Neil Bush and the Savings and Loan? And how that scandal of George Bush's son parallels the Bailey Building and Loan?"

"Shhh," they whispered in unison. There was no time for a social studies lesson during Christmas vacation. School was out!

My daughters had ganged up on me again and were in the separate sister world that they seemed to inhabit; when they were younger and wanted to exclude me by speaking gibberish. When they spoke their own special language I felt as powerless as a Japanese code breaker trying to decipher Navajo during World War II. Sometimes I think the two of them were actually twins for they were as close as the identical twins, Jenni and Beth.

And today Courtney and I talk about Taylor, and Courtney claims to channel her sister and sometimes I feel the same, especially when I'm driving the Tercel with her rosary beads on the stick shift, which are there more to comfort me now than as remembrance of things past. I hear a *Hi, Pops*, in my mind. Then Taylor and I are back watching George Bailey once again, sharing a bowl of microwave popcorn. *It Was a Wonderful Life, wasn't it?*

* * *

After the mad dash to the airport and the return trip to South Florida, Taylor and I prepared for a return to Duke and the stem cell harvest. The idea was to take some of Taylor's stem cells and freeze them and then use them after chemotherapy to bring back her immunity system. I was never comfortable with chemotherapy for it seemed illogical to treat cancer by injecting toxins into a patient's body, but I certainly didn't claim to have a better idea.

Taylor's Diary
January 30, 2001

Today I get a Broviac Hickman port installed (at least that's what I think it is). What it is is annoying. It is two 6 inch tubes hanging out of my chest. They use it for the stem cell harvest, so it will only be in for a week or so. Thank heavens!

Anyway, it was an outpatient surgery so it only took a couple of hours, which is always a plus. Other than that I just hung out w/Karly and Gia awhile and got caught up. It was nice. And then the munchkins came by. Kristine (Taylor's sister-in-law and mother of her little nieces) asked me to be Godmother for Anya which, of course, I happily accepted. Then later in the evening Katie and Karly came

68

over and we just talked for a couple of hours. In all it was (besides the "procedure") a very comforting day.

Apparently I go back to N.C. on Thursday and I have to stay up there until next Fri.! I'm not sure how long of down time I have between that and my migration to Gainesville (we arranged for radiation to be given at the University of Florida's Shands Hospital with sister Courtney becoming the caretaker). Hopefully a couple of days. I'm really not gonna see Jeff much for a long while and on top of that right after graduation he is moving to North Carolina, so I guess we'll take it from there. I don't really have much to say about life, except maybe that I'm not very insightful. On another note, I am getting very frustrated w/myself because it always seems that there are the little things that I mean to do that slip through my fingers day after day.

Am I that much of a flake? I am starting to get fed up w/the whole "cancer" thing. (Strange as it may sound). I'm getting annoyed w/doctors, hospitals, antibiotics, needles and so forth. This is a problem because I know if I let myself become bothered by all of it then it will only make the time absolutely wretched. So, I must consciously (sp?) keep a positive outlook. I mean there are worse things in life. This is only a brief period. Always remember that!

Two days later Taylor and I were off to Duke. The National Children's Cancer Society secured a room for us in Durham at the University Inn, across the street from the Duke Hospital. The National Children's Cancer Society helped families at Duke and other hospitals and the cost savings were a Godsend.

Most HMOs wouldn't cover stem cell harvesting, so it was a good thing that Taylor had a PPO insurance policy with Celtic for Kids out of Chicago, which turned out to be a great insurance company. The last thing a parent wanted was an insurance company to deny coverage to his child for a procedure which might save her life.

The McGovern Children's Hospital at Duke was a kid-friendly place with an open air design and see-through elevators—mobiles right out of the Calder catalogue. Orange, red and yellow flower mobiles hang from the ceiling.

There was an Islamic woman in a veil seeking help and speaking, appropriately, Arabic. People come from all over the world to be treated at Duke because of a Dr. Kurtzberg and her work on fetal cord blood.

But we were there for "pheresis" as stem cell harvesting is known. The medical technician took cells out of the patient's body, froze them and then returned the rest of the blood back to the patient. Taylor was instructed to bring plenty of Tums for the calcium in the tablets helps with the discomfort of letting one's blood be sucked out and recycled.

And then the game plan post pheresis was that Taylor would receive radiation for six weeks and then a transplant which would require 28-45 days at Duke in isolation as she would have run the risk of infection for 3-6 months.

Taylor sat in a room with a teenage boy from Cleveland, who was suffering from medulloblastoma, as both of them were having their blood drawn out. She read from *Harry Potter and the Goblet of Fire*. Thank God for Hogwarts. At least Taylor was able to escape into J.K. Rowlings's fantasy world.

Taylor's Diary
February 3, 2001

I write to you from the icy land of Durham. Yes, my father and I have come for the stem cell harvest (pheresis). Well, that takes place on Mon., Wed and Fri., for about 3 hrs. or more a piece. I have to sit in a room while they collect my stem cells.

(I have to get my Nupogen for the first 3 days prior and then all the week of pheresis).

So, other than that we are pretty much free which I love, disliking hospitals so much and all. But, wouldn't you know me? I have to go and have low hemoglobin which means I have to get a blood transfusion before the whole procedure. I did that today. In there I met a very nice guy named Tristan. He has medulloblastoma (brain tumor found in the base of your head by the brain stem). His had also spread to his spine. He was diagnosed in the Jan. before this and since has undergone chemo and radiation, two rounds of pheresis and is currently undergoing more chemo. He was very good natured. Hopefully I'll see him around. I hope w/all my heart that he beats it.

Other than that things have been pretty dull here. I've been doing a lot of reading and getting lost w/Dad trying to find simple places. Tracey Dawn and Cindy are coming tomorrow, so that should be some entertainment.

Well, I've been here for 3 days but I still got a week to go and already I miss Jeff tremendously. I hope we can last through all the separation, but what do they say: "absences makes the heart grow fonder." Hopefully, but they also say, "outta sight, outta mind."

So I get back home next Sat. the 10th and hopefully I'll have a few days before I have to go up to Shands. But that shouldn't be too bad. Well, poor Dad, he's such an early bird I think I've been disrupting his sleep because I'm up so late. On that note, I think I'll retire.

Chapter Fourteen: I Guess It Doesn't Matter Anymore

As I was driving the Tercel today, I tossed in a Buddy Holly cassette—yes, I still have cassettes—and listened as the legend of Lubbock crooned *I Guess It Doesn't Matter Anymore,* and thought back to an incident with Taylor when I stupidly continued to be a teacher rather than a father.

A week after Taylor's first brain surgery I took a day off from school to drive Taylor to Martin County High School so she could turn in a paper in a dual enrollment class. Dual enrollment classes were classes taught through Indian River Community College, but on the high school campuses. I taught two dual enrollment classes at my school, South Fork High School, Martin County's rival. So we walked onto campus so she could turn in an English paper. A week after surgery and she was walking with a limp, for God's sake. Surely a brain tumor would have been a good enough reason to turn a paper in late, but I encouraged her to get it done and turn it in. God, looking back on it, I was just like my father who forced me to play football from 7th through 12th grade even though I was a geek on the gridiron, a benchwarmer, who, during the games generally played "left out" instead of left tackle. My father had been a good football player in both high school and college and I was his last hope, being the last son he sired. Oldest brother Mike had lasted two days of high school practice, having had the good luck to obtain a concussion and consequently a 4-F for football; brother Tom, who was always able to find a way out of things and would thus go on to a successful business career, literally and figuratively ran away from football by lettering in cross country. So it was up to me to fulfill my father's fantasies of a son winning the Heisman Trophy. I resented my father for the football obsession, and there I was, forcing Taylor, after brain surgery no less, to turn in the silly English paper, which Taylor later informed me she had finished under pain killers. My rationale was I had to continue to be my teacher self in encouraging her to turn the paper in. Any deviation in my behavior and Taylor might sense I didn't think she was going to beat this "brain cancer thing." That's the way I honestly felt, and looking back, that was really a rationalization for me, part of my own denial; I was terrified that Taylor was *not* going to beat this "brain cancer thing" and I coped with it through her courage, not my own.

As Taylor, wearing a blue bandana head covering that would become her trademark, hobbled across the campus that day to turn in her paper, I stood stoically like the idiotic pedagogue I could be, contemplating that no student in my classes would ever have a reason for turning in a paper late if my own daughter with a brain tumor had turned her paper in on time.

And as Taylor turned the corner and limped out of sight down a hallway, I began to cry. Hell, I didn't just cry, I blubbered like a baby, sobbing for several seconds before I regained control of my emotions. I was relieved that no one saw me as all of the students and teachers were in class. I was proud of Taylor and wondered where she got her guts. Obviously not from her crybaby father, I remember thinking. She probably got her guts from her mother. I remember thinking that my ex-wife Pam was a tough old bird, I'd give her that.

Within a week, Taylor's girlfriends were wearing bandanas in sympathy for Taylor. It was a touching show of friendship which caught on among the senior girls and became a fashion statement at the oh so preppy Martin County High School.

Looking at Taylor's journal now, I noticed an entry from October 18th 2000, about ten days after she turned in the English paper. It was that poem, reproduced earlier about the doctor's "sad look upon our face."

As it turned out Taylor received a C+ on that paper which she considered a gift considering she typed the paper's last paragraph three times due to the influence of the Percocet.

I later apologized to Taylor for pressing her so hard about the English paper but she forgave me and laughed about it. Looking back I was sorry I was such a hard ass, but when I beat myself up, I think of Taylor as a little girl, sitting in the passenger seat of the Tercel as we shoot up Interstate 95 to Pennsylvania and Nana-land and Buddy Holly is on and Taylor is singing slightly off-key in that tiny little voice: *I Guess It Doesn't Matter*

* * *

Meanwhile, back in Durham, North Carolina, things didn't go as smoothly as planned with pheresis....

Taylor's Diary
February 7, 2001

I know I haven't kept update info about the whole pheresis. I guess subconsciously (and even perhaps consciously) I didn't want to think about it. But, just to update everything now, here's what happened. I went in on Mon. and started out fine. Then about 30 mins. into it I got a blood clot in my line. It took 2 hrs. for pharmacy to bring TPA (the stuff they use to unclot it) and then you have to wait for a half an hr., so we decided to do it the next day (yesterday). Well, about 45 mins. into yesterday the technician takes a closer look at my line and brings in a nurse technician. They discover that the "wonderful" people down @ St. Mary's put in the wrong line. So, now I have surgery tom. To put in the right line. I can't even tell you how much anger and frustration I was filled w/ and still partially filled w/ Now, I am not projected to leave here until the middle of next week sometime. If all goes well I may be able to go on Mon. night or Tues. And then supposedly I only have a day or two before I go to Shands (the University of Florida's hospital in Gainesville). This is the most upsetting for me because @home I rebuild my strength (at least psychologically). Also, this means I will only get to see Jeff for about a day before I got off for 6 weeks. I don't know. I guess I'm just really bummed because of the whole situation, and I'm really trying to look on the bright side of things because I honestly believe that negative thinking will make the situation worse. I tell myself this but then in all reality how long can you really be away from an attractive guy whose always having fun and being around girls before he wonders why he is holding on to you anyway. After all, you are just a phone girlfriend with the rare occasion of seeing him for a day or two maybe twice a month. What do I do if the probable comes to fruition? I don't know if I'll be able to bear it. He has been my strength in ways that others could not. I suppose in the meantime I can only hope that does not happen and cross that bridge when I come to it. For now though I will try to be optimistic.

P.S. Dad and I are going to a basketball game w/Friedman tom. night—to see Georgia play.

Chapter Fifteen: Love Is Infinite

I have a friend who used the term "I released him to his future" when talking about an employee she decided to let go, and I adopted the phrase when I referred to my divorce, that my wife didn't divorce me but rather that she released me to my future, a future of sobriety, solvency and sanity. But one day, when Taylor was in the seventh grade, a year of worry and wonder when the hormonal changes of early adolescence were set on high, we sat at the kitchen table while Taylor nibbled away at a buttered baked potato. Suddenly, she suggested, "let's go to Shepard's Park and see the sunset, Dad."

Taylor loved sunrises and sunsets, the alpha and the omegas of the day. I'm sure if she had been an Egyptian girl three or four thousand years ago she would have been a Ra Ra, a cheerleader for the sun god. It is interesting when children are small that they see more sunrises than sunsets, but it reverses itself in adolescence for teens prefer the sunset to the sunrise.

Shepard's Park was a great place for a sunset and I agreed to take Taylor there, for I enjoyed the walkway out over the river. That day the St. Lucie River was tranquil as usual. Small boats with "liveaboads" were rocking gently, anchored against languorous current. Across the river the sun was beginning to dip down over Palm City. It was a postcard p.m. Taylor felt chatty.

"Dad, something weird happened in school today," Taylor began.

I asked her to explain.

"A new girl in class."

"Okay, so?"

"Dad, her parents live together," Taylor said.

I chuckled. Was that it?

"What's so funny, Dad?"

Seeing the perplexed look on her face, I recall I erased my smile and asked her to go on with her story.

"Well we all gathered around her and asked her what it was like to have two parents on your case all the time."

Then it hit me. Most of Taylor's friends came from "broken homes," as my mother used to call them: children of divorce. Children from two parent families were anomalies to Taylor and her friends, except Mike and Pat Jordan. Since Pam had "released me to my future" when Taylor was only five, she didn't remember when Pam and I had lived together.

I remembered saying something witty in response to her, something like. "Hard to divide and conquer when the parents are under the same roof, eh?"

"Yeah." She responded.

"Are you sorry Mom and I aren't together, Taylor?"

"Heck no," she said with a smile I considered a bit too mischievous. "I like it better this way."

Which I knew translated into: I can get away with anything at Mom's. Her mother had a more laisseze-faire attitude toward child rearing, but after seven children perhaps her child raising might have been viewed more or less as a survival tactic.

"But the new girl…" Taylor went on, "it was as strange that her situation wasn't normal for my group of friends. Most kids go back between a mom and a dad. That's what seems right to us." She thought for a moment and then changed the subject, "The sunset is pretty isn't it, Daddy?"

It was what the ad man might have dubbed "a Kodak moment," father and daughter admiring the sundown together, but there was no photographer to snap a picture for posterity. I wish there had been. And she called me "Daddy."

"Daddy!" She hadn't called me "Daddy" in quite some time. I put my arm around her shoulder and smiled as the sun went down.

"I love you, Taylor," I said.

"I love you as much as infinity," she replied, and for the next couple of years she would add infinity to her love. When I think of her sisters with their infinity tattoos I am reminded of Taylor's "I love you infinity, Daddy."

And now she is with infinity, with the Alpha and the Omega, her day is done, her sun has set and she is with The Son. She is with the Infinite. It was a divine calling.

Taylor's Diary
February 8, 2001

Today I had surgery for the new line. Let's hope this is the right one. (It was). My chest is still sore but, that is to be expected. I slept for a few hrs. in the afternoon and then Dad & I went to a basketball game w/Friedman to see Georgia (Georgia Schweitzer was the star of the Duke Women's Basketball Team and would go on to the W.N.B.A.). She was great, but unfortunately they lost to FSU by 2 pts. A really unexpected outcome to the game. After that I went to 5200 (the isolation ward at Duke Hospital, made possible by a gift by Perry Como and his wife) to get my shot. I believe the nurses are getting frustrated that I have to keep going there for it. (Because her father was a wimp who couldn't bear to stick a needle in his daughter's arm). But, Beth's coming Sat. so hopefully we can get some GCSF so she can give it to me here. Well, it's been a week since we arrived and it feels like eternity. But, I guess I better change my mindset cause I'm gonna be here awhile longer. Jeez, I don't know what I'm gonna do when I have to stay a month. I met a woman tonight (on the floor) whose precious little daughter has cancer; it's been in remission now for 15 months. She was telling me about her daughter's diagnosis and treatment and all she had been through. God bless her! Children, especially very young children, that have to go through this ordeal are without a doubt angels. There is no other way they would be able to prevail. From what I have seen in the brief time I have been experiencing this (compared to others) there are definitely many angels here on earth.

It was a sad day for me two days later when I had to wake Taylor to accompany me to the airport. I had to get back to work. My job was essential as I had to pay for the insurance. Sister Beth was relieving me.

Beth and her twin sister Jenni had been very close to me. I met them at age 3 and they were my daughters (technically stepdaughters) from age 3 to 12. When Pam and I divorced, she cut off my contact with the twins. But Beth had moved back home and I made a phone call and helped her get an interview for a teaching position; Taylor's illness had a positive effect in one sense as I was able to see the twins again. Beth had sent me an "amends" letter, apologizing for the way

I was treated. She had been out on a date and her date bought her a York Peppermint Patty and she burst out crying, because that was the candy I bought her and Jenni after school when she was a little girl. A flood of memories engulfed her: her loss. My loss. Jenni would send an "amends" letter as well.

Anyway, as Taylor and I waited for Beth to fly in and me to fly out, I felt like a deserter. My daughter was crying. The medical screw-ups forced Taylor to stay longer and for me to return. And Beth to ride to the rescue.

When Beth appeared, Taylor turned the faucet off, but I still felt guilty.

Chapter Sixteen: Are They Filming a St. Jude's Commercial?

After Taylor's first brain surgery we were referred to the St. Mary's Pediatric Oncology Unit in West Palm Beach to begin chemotherapy. In retrospect I wonder if Taylor should have received radiation treatment before chemotherapy but the protocol was determined by Dr. Henry Friedman at Duke University, and even though I would receive a post *60 Minutes* letter from Taylor's original neurosurgeon, Dr. Michael Paul, questioning the treatment, in 2011 the whole discussion is rather moot. After all, it was Dr. Paul who recommended the cancer team at St. Mary's, and they steered us to Duke, and Duke oversaw the treatment.

My first impression of St. Mary's Pediatric Oncology floor that first day was that I was in the middle of a St. Jude's Hospital commercial, sans violin music, and I thought at any moment Marlo Thomas or some has-been TV actor or a D-list celebrity would pop out into the hospital corridor with a canister, pleading for a contribution. Was this what hell was like? Bald children? To a parent, bald children can be more frightening than all of Dante's circles of perdition.

But you wouldn't have known this was hell from the kids.

Tiny tots with their eyes all aglow were not having trouble sleeping, they were navigating the floor, rolling their aluminum stands with the IV bottles attached. Playing videogames! Listening to music. Smiling and laughing. What was wrong with them? Were they oblivious? *Maybe not,* I thought. Don't they have cancer? Shouldn't they be in their beds worrying about dying? Like grownups would? Of course, there was no need for background violin music or Marlo and her guilt-trip groupies, for these kids pulled at your heartstrings without the need of orchestration or a voice-over.

I couldn't walk down the corridor without getting a lump in my throat. Here were the hopes and dreams of so many families, the boys and girls of today who had been sidetracked on their journeys to become men and women of tomorrow. Many wouldn't make it to voting age, their first beer, or even to a driver's license or a senior prom. And yet they were cheery-faced, happy with this day, living in the moment, truly living in the "Now" as my twelve-step program preaches. This was a place where children stayed and it wasn't hell at all, it was hope, and it was staffed by those everyday heroes, the floor nurses, women who were overworked and underpaid. Doctors were often haughty, nurses had heart. Why was it nurses aren't more appreciated?

Pam, Taylor, Courtney and I met with the "team," a group of doctors, nurses and social workers. There was a blackboard with the chalk outline of a skull. Welcome to Brain Cancer 101 and the cancer classroom. Please find a seat. Dr. MacArthur drew a brain inside the chalk outline of a skull to show us the location of Taylor's tumor and listed the negatives of chemotherapy.

Leukemia as a side effect! That's pretty friggin' negative!

I don't remember much after that little "side effect" although I did perk up when Dr. MacArthur mentioned "sterility." *God*, I thought, *she will contract leukemia and wind up sterile. Hell, let's have chemotherapy, it really sounds like a winner to me.* The doctor then asked, "Are there any questions?"

I remember asking, "What *good* does chemotherapy do?"

"It kills the tumor," the doctor replied, looking at me as if I were an imbecile. And in fact, I was an imbecile, at least when it came to brain cancer. But we would learn the chemotherapy didn't do any good, not in all of its various forms. And in the end, Taylor realized the inefficacy of chemotherapy and refused to have any more of it, for the only thing it did was make her nauseous. Today a friend of mine, suffering from cancer, told me there have been great advances since 2001, but I still wonder. The concept of killing something by poisoning the patient's body makes no logical sense to this layman.

I know I am not a physician and don't claim to be all that bright, but I keep thinking perhaps that someday someone will look back on chemotherapy as we now look at the practice of bloodletting. Benjamin Rush, the most prominent American physician in the late 18th century, was a great believer in "bleeding," but I would be deathly afraid to go to Dr. Rush today for treatment.

I would have a different opinion of chemotherapy had it worked for Taylor and in the end of her life the doctors were administering the same form of chemotherapy which had failed in the first month of treatment. And what I have learned about the definition of insanity is: trying the same thing over and over and expecting different results.

Surgery worked as far as that goes. Radiation slowed the tumor down, but chemotherapy turned out to be a bust.

Two weeks before she died, I had to intervene on Taylor's behalf as the oncologist at Martin Memorial continued the chemotherapy protocol which was still on her charts even though they had an incorrect diagnosis of medulloblastoma.

"Dad," Taylor said to me, looking to me for help. "I don't want any more chemo. It doesn't work and it just makes me sick."

I knew I had to do something, anything to help her. "Okay, Taylor," I said and called the nurse in. I remember that moment as if were this morning.

"Nurse," I said. "Taylor is 18, of legal age, and she has something to say that I want you to put in the chart. Go ahead Taylor."

"No more chemo. It just makes me sick," Taylor said angrily from her hospital bed.

"Will you please note her wishes on her chart, nurse?"

"Yes sir," the nurse said.

And from that moment on, for the brief remainder of her life, Taylor never took chemotherapy again.

* * *

After the pheresis at Duke, Taylor would make it back to Stuart in time for Valentine's Day. Ever the hopeless romantic, Taylor had a few short days home before she had to go off to Gainesville for radiation.

Taylor's Diary
February 14, 2001

Happy Valentine's Day!

Actually, this has been the worst V-Day ever. But we'll get to that later, first I will catch you up on the past week. Dad was relieved of duty by Beth and Tracy C., Tracey Dawn and Cindy all came into town. It was rather an enjoyable weekend. Then we wrapped up the pheresis on Mon.& Tues. and came back last night. So, at least I'm home awhile until I have to go back to Gainesville which will probably be Mon. So, the latest news of my love life or lack thereof; let me just start by saying Jeff & I broke up.

To go into further detail: At the end of my trip (the last couple of days) Jeff was being strange every time I talked to him and even didn't answer my calls one night. So, I didn't tell him I came back into town but then decided to call him on Valentine's Day. So I called, of course, he didn't answer, seeing the caller ID. And then later I left a message saying that we needed to talk. He called me back and asked if he could come over and was really acting strange. So I looked him in the eye and asked if he had cheated on me. He laughed and said he knew I was going to ask him that. The answer was "no," then I said, "Do you just want to date me?" He gave a stuttering answer saying, "Well, no it's not that, but I feel guilty talking to you when I'm with my friends and it's like I have a girlfriend but I don't because you're never here and I never get to see you."

This would all be understood and forgivable if it had not been for one thing. I told him several times in the very beginning not to date me because it wasn't fair to him and this would ultimately happen. He told me time and again that he could handle it, he was sure, and that it wouldn't be a problem. After a lot of resistance on my part he finally persuaded me that he would see this through no matter what. This is the reason that I am so hurt and this is the reason I no longer will have him in any part of my life. He swore to me time and again that he could handle it and be loyal and faithful and then he goes and does the one thing I begged him not do in the first place. I feel absolutely awful inside and I

87

still want him. But, I have to be strong and move on. I am not going to make that a cycle. So, there goes Jeff gone from my life forever after a few curt words and a very heated argument. He is no more. He is only a figment of my imagination of something that might have once been, a very long time ago. With that I trudge forward, dropping him like dirty laundry. Already I feel lighter. My heart is a little heavy, but my load has lightened some.

Like most seventeen-year-olds Taylor could be overly dramatic. The "forever" wouldn't last, of course, and her relationship with Jeff would resume. It was difficult enough being a teenager. A teen was insecure and self-conscious. Throw cancer into the mix and a kid really had a struggle.

Chapter Seventeen: Timothy Trump

I was cleaning out the laundry room the other day and came upon the battered cardboard box of *Monopoly*. It had been sitting unused on a shelf for years, gathering dust and it seemed, holding fast to a memory, for as I opened the game there was Taylor's playing piece which she invariably chose: the little dog. I was a "top hat" man myself: I wondered if I chose the top hat in memory of Bobby Freimuth, a boy with whom I had played a hundred *Monopoly* games the summer after he lost his leg to cancer.

Springfield, Pennsylvania, 1962. The Cuban Missile Crisis would come that fall and the world would sit, teetering, one harsh word from nuclear Armageddon, but in the summer of 1962, the summer in which *American Graffiti* is set, one-legged Bobby Freimuth would hobble around the neighborhood on his crutches to play a game of *Monopoly* with me. He would die in the spring of 1963, a victim of metastasis as the cancer spread throughout his body. I think Taylor was perhaps eleven when I told her the story of Bobby Freimuth during a game of *Monopoly*. How could I know that I would tell the story of Bobby's cancer to a daughter who would later contract the disease as well?

I was showing Taylor no mercy in the game; I never did. Still, she was eager to play; she was always willing to play games with me. I would play chess with Taylor and remove my rooks until she got better and I removed only one. Then one day she beat me at chess with my one rook removed and that was the last time I removed a rook. She didn't beat me after that but she was able to beat every boy at J.D. Parker Elementary and that was empowering: beating boys was where it was at in elementary school. That attitude about boys would certainly change!

But in *Monopoly*, she was a disaster. There was no room in *Monopoly* for an empathetic capitalist. Whoever heard of such a creature? She should have been confined to the low rent properties like Baltic Avenue. If Taylor were ahead in the game she'd let Courtney skip rent when her sister landed on her properties, but, on the other hand, she would never give me a free pass. I guess you might say her empathy was selective. Still, she seemed to have bad luck at *Monopoly*, and that particular day I owned Boardwalk and Park Place and had built hotels on each property. Taylor was already frustrated when she rolled the dice and landed on Boardwalk.

I grabbed the Boardwalk deed gleefully and read the bad news to her. "With a hotel, that is two thousand dollars you owe me, Taylor." Then I added in my best Wicked Witch of the West voice, pointing to her canine-shaped playing piece. "And I want your little dog too!"

Taylor glared and me and looked at her paltry pile of play money. "I don't have the money, Timothy Trump."

I laughed at the nickname. That was pretty good, I thought. "You want a loan?"

"No," she replied with a resigned look on her face. "I lost. You beat me, Timothy Trump."

The teacher in me took over at that point. "You know, Taylor, calling me Trump is perfect as this whole game board was designed on the basis of Atlantic City and Donald Trump has a casino there."

"I know, Dad, you told me a million times."

"Oh," I remember saying.

Her eyes twinkled and she retorted. "Old people repeat themselves, don't they Dad?"

"You think I'm old?"

"Not too old...just old enough," she smiled.

I wasn't done my teaching for the day, however. "You know you need to develop your properties, Taylor. When you get a set of properties you need to build houses and hotels. Build, build, build. That's how I win."

"I don't care if I win, Dad," I remember she replied. "I just want to spend time with you. I liked the story about your friend, Dad, the boy who died of cancer and the games you played with him. I think of that boy and winning doesn't seem very important. You spent time with Bobby, that was important. I mean he couldn't play sports anymore and the other boys ignored him. Just spending time together seems important. Dad, you told me the top hat was his piece and you use it every time we play. Nana said you even wrote a poem about him. Do you remember when I was little and I told everyone I wasn't going to be here long?"

Yes, I remembered *that* then and I remember it now. Taylor was perhaps four or five when she told everyone that she wasn't going to be around long. Did she know that somehow as a little child? Did her soul know a secret? I remember telling Taylor that yes, I did remember what she said when she was young. Then we put away the *Monopoly* box and for the next month or so, when we played the game, I was dubbed Timothy Trump. I came across the poem for Bobby a while back; my mother had kept it, and thrown out all of my baseball cards of course. I might be rich now, if it had been the other way around. But then so would every other man my age, whose mother cleaned out her attic and tossed out his childhood treasures. If I still had my Mickey Mantle and Willie Mays cards, even the creased one that I stuck in my bike spokes, maybe then I could have been a real Timothy Trump. But then, memories are more precious than money aren't they?

* * *

After a few days at home, Taylor was off to Gainesville and radiation. She moved in with Courtney in her apartment and Courtney took the semester off so she could oversee Taylor's radiation treatment. A big responsibility for a twenty-year-old to look after her eighteen-year-old sister? Taylor was closer to Courtney than to anyone and even at twenty Courtney was the most level-headed of seven children.

Taylor's Diary
February 20, 2001

Well, I am now in Gainesville. So far it promises to be a pleasurable experience (much more pleasurable than Duke). Everything w/Jeff is still up in the air. He came over the night before I left 'till about 4 in the morning. He is really hot and cold and I don't know what he wanted from me. So I suppose for now I should just put him out of my mind. Yes, that's what I'll do. Anyway, I don't know if I'm going home this weekend, it seems as though no one is going. So, I went to Shands today and had a consultation, MRI and a mold done. I have to go back in Thurs. for a CT scan. But my MRI had a clean scan so that's awesome. See the things I get excited about now? Sometimes I think about my life a year ago. I was going through w/o a care in the world. It seems like a lifetime ago. Everything is so different now and everyone in my life has become something different to me.

Taylor's Diary
February 21, 2001

So I am going home this weekend (tomorrow actually) which is good because otherwise I wouldn't be able to go for like 3 weeks. I hope there is stuff to do this weekend though you know what I was just thinking? Every day we wander the earth with billions of other people and so many different lives. It just makes you think, doesn't it? Of the infinite possibilities and the millions of different ways people choose to live their lives. Which is the way I should choose to live mine? I suppose it'll come along piece by piece. I think it's just reminding yourself everyday to drop everything and look around and really notice the beauty in nature and in the world and all its people. I watched the sun shine through leaves today and it lifted me.

Chapter Eighteen: Reefer Saneness

I come across Taylor's poems in her journals and in old shoe boxes now and again, and they often take me back to the last year of her life as many of them deal with her illness and her response to the cancer.

> *The anticipation of disease is a bitch no one should know.*
> *The waiting is like a rollercoaster with the severest low.*
> *Day in day out the same, no news has yet been heard,*
> *And so the time will pass as we wait to learn the word.*
> *A doctor here, a hospital there, to me it's all the same*
> *For now I just sit waiting for the day that I go lame.*
> *My body bruised and beaten will surely quit somehow,*
> *Until that day I'll wait and pray for when that time is now.*

Of course that 'now' did come and prior to her death she did go nearly lame, but that year had its amusing moments as well, when Taylor's siblings rallied around her and beat the system in what I like to refer to as "reefer saneness." Marijuana, it seems, was the one thing she could count on to counteract the nausea of chemotherapy.

Most people are too young to have heard of the classic Depression era anti-marijuana propaganda film *Reefer Madness* that warned of the evils of pot. That was during the time when prohibition was being repealed and booze was flowing legally once again in the United States. Marijuana was a possible competitor to booze, and the liquor lobby was successful in having pot declared an illegal narcotic. Ironically, unlike alcohol which causes nausea, the THC in marijuana has anti-nausea properties which are helpful to chemotherapy patients. The medical establishment had no trouble prescribing pot pills for Taylor to relieve her nausea, but unfortunately they were

1) Ridiculously expensive and 2) completely worthless. The secret to nausea relief was in the delivery system. Relief from chemo nausea required the express lane of the lungs, not the traffic jam on the backed up digestive system, and only smoking the pot accomplished that.

Taylor was on court-ordered probation for the Possum Long Pot caper of the summer before and, I suppose, theoretically, a judge might have sent her to the slammer for smoking a bit of weed, but even a law-abiding high school teacher could see the folly of Florida's marijuana laws. Yet in 2001, the progressive state of California hadn't passed its medical marijuana statutes, and one might say that the whole nation was suffering from a bit of reefer madness in its prohibition of pot for medicinal purposes. Heck, even the ancient conservative senator from South Carolina, Strom Thurmond, believed pot should be legalized for medical treatment.

Taylor had just had a session of some really nasty chemotherapy at St. Mary's in West Palm Beach and was constantly making trips from her hospital bed to the bathroom to barf in the room's toilet, dragging her IV stand beside her. It was, as she said, "a regular barfarama."

"I need pot, Dad," I remember she said to me, tears in her eyes. Vomiting was not her favorite pastime.

"I know," I replied, feeling totally powerless.

"Dammit," she cursed. "Shit!"

Taylor was really feeling bad. It wasn't that she was a saint and didn't swear, she just didn't swear around me. At least not often. "I'm sorry for swearing, Dad," she apologized.

"Don't worry about it, honey," I replied and gave her a hug. "Sometimes swearing is necessary."

And then a white knight appeared. Taylor's sibling, who shall remain nameless due to the statute of limitations, came to visit bringing oranges, citrus spray, a small fan, and…weed.

"Tim, guard the door," the sibling told me. He opened the hospital room window and moved near the opening. Taylor sat in the chair, lit the pipe and exhaled the smoke out the window as the fan circulated citrus smell throughout the room. The oranges, I realized, were the "cover" fruit. Florida's top two cash crops, pot and oranges, were involved. I suppose I could rationalize that we were doing our civic duty, but in my mind I saw Anita Bryant, who had once been the spokesperson for the orange industry, smoking a joint and that didn't work.

"Make sure the nurses don't come in, Tim," the sibling ordered me and I went out and guarded the door to the room, promising to signal with the secret family knock if a nurse neared. Meanwhile, in the hospital room, Taylor puffed away her nausea with the sibling-provided pot. For the first time in my life I was thankful for the substance abuse in the family. I wondered for a moment if my marriage might have worked with marijuana in lieu of alcohol, but I will never know. Still it was a remarkable family that could come up with pot in a tight spot, at a moment's notice. Our folks could obtain the tokes, one might say.

Of course outside the door standing guard, my imagination got the best of me and I envisioned a headline in the *Stuart News*: "Local Teacher Serves as Lookout for Pot Head Daughter." And my mind began to write the copy in the

5 W journalistic format (who, what, when, where, and why) which I had taught my journalism students back in the '80s.

But that night I truly changed my opinion on the use of marijuana for cancer patients, because I saw how pot worked for Taylor. I can hear her voice in my head now, laughing about the whole incident.

You were so nervous, you were funny, Pops. We had everything under control. The fan, the citrus. You were dealing with professionals, Pops. There weren't many funny times in that year, but that was one of them. *There I was sticking my head out of the hospital room window, blowing pot smoke into the air.* Taylor appreciated the irony of being on probation for pot. To her it was a hoot.

I wish there had been more moments like that.

* * *

Looking back on that year of Taylor's treatment, I think that radiation prolonged her life. Although it didn't rid her of the tumor, in the end it slowed its growth and gave her perhaps a few more months. Still, at the beginning, like the eternal optimists that we had become, we thought perhaps that radiation would save her. We were wrong.

Taylor's Diary
March 2, 2001

I have started radiation. It is not a fun experience let me tell you. The first day I came home w/a headache and severe case of vomiting. After I smoked a little bit (marijuana) I was fine and able to hold down food. I am going to ask Friedman if he has any objections to that.

Taylor's Diary
March 4, 2001

I have consciously been avoiding writing in this journal. I'm not sure why; only I think it may be because I've entered another stage of this epiphany. I haven't really grasped what I am supposed to have learned from this. I believe I have learned that life is a miracle, every second of it. But I don't think I have the outlook all the time. I at least want to see it that way more days than not.

Taylor's Diary
March 8, 2001

Radiation has been wearing me down a bit. I sleep a lot and I am fatigued throughout the day when the actual radiation is taking place. I have the strange sensation and then the most horrible smell overwhelms me. It smells like burning flesh or something disgustingly similar to that. I'm going to try and get my appt. moved up to tom. because we're gonna go home.

Chapter Nineteen: My So-Called Life

Watching a rerun of one of Taylor's favorite TV programs, *My So Called Life,* a television show about a fifteen-year-old coping with adolescence, I was browsing through one of Taylor's old journals and her list of New Year's resolutions for 1998, the year she turned fifteen. After watching the program it seemed appropriate.

I resolve to:

1. *stop caring what other people think*
2. *listen to myself more than anyone else*
3. *stop being ultra-sensitive but still sensitive*
4. *get over my petty problems and focus on other people, not myself*
5. *set goals and achieve them*
6. *stick to things when I say I'll do them*
7. *not be such a flake*
8. *learn self-control and will power*
9. *not be so afraid of getting hurt*
10. *open up more, but only to a select few, communicate more*

Looking back on her resolutions, I thought it was a good list, but of course we are humans and we are flawed, and when you are fifteen and find Erik, nothing else seems to matter. 1998 was not the year of the rat or dog, it was the Year of the Erik. Erik, Erik! He wasn't Erik the Red, he was Erik the Loser, but he was her first real boyfriend and nothing is as blinding as one's first infatuation, even if he has an acne problem.

Of course at the time, like most fathers, I didn't know the depth of her feeling for Erik the L and coming across a diary entry of July 6, 1998 I found:

My boyfriend Erik is perhaps one of the greatest people I have met though he does have his flaws. Although I do seem to have some type of relationship phobia (I know this coming from a 15 yr. old must sound ridiculous)

No, Taylor, I thought as I reread it: It didn't sound ridiculous at all. It sounded human. It was honest. We have all had those feeling, honey; I wish I could have told her then. But we didn't talk about Erik very much; Taylor was more distant at fifteen, into the world of peer pressure and, on occasion, bad choices. Erik the L was certainly a bad choice and by September he had been arrested for possession of marijuana.

"Erik got busted for pot, Dad," she told me one evening.

Little did I know that for Taylor it was a preview of coming attractions in her own life.

I was sitting at the kitchen table hiding behind a newspaper. That was one of my father's best tactics when I was an adolescent. My father didn't want to show the anger he felt when, as a teenager, I would say something to piss him off, like informing him I was going to skip college to go hop with the kangaroos in Australia because I didn't want to be part of a country that was at war in Vietnam. It was calculated, of course, for I was far too big a coward to hightail it down under and wound up at the good Lutheran school, Gettysburg College. Funny, how we learn things from our parents. "That's too bad," I said, but I wasn't angry, I was feeling guiltily grateful. Perhaps this was the end of the reign of Erik the L. Perhaps he would sail off to the New World and rediscover

Newfoundland, Nova Scotia or a new Starbucks on South Beach.

"Looks like I won't be seeing him for a while," Taylor said. She didn't seem all that broken up about it, as I recall. I knew she was waiting for my reaction.

Yes! I thought and, certain my smile was erased, brought down my newspaper. It was a signal; Taylor went on as if making her closing argument to a judge. If it may please my father's court: She didn't enter an oral argument that night, but rather wrote in her journal:

I know Erik may sound like a lose, but he's the farthest thing from it. He's such a great person. I hope that when I look back on this I'll remember all those little things that made him so noble and good.

But within a week, Erik the L was in the past.

* * *

My first great love was a girl name Lynda who, I remember, had a great swimming pool. But today when I try to envision Lynda's face, all I get is the pool. I assume she went on to marry someone and have children and so forth, but I really only remember the summer I spent in her swimming pool. Lynda the Pool, I guess, or simply Lynda the P. It was a nice, kidney shaped pool in a Philadelphia suburb and I skipped a summer typing class nearly every day to be near Lynda the P. A cool dip in a girl's pool certainly beat the hum of an IBM *Selectric* typewriter. I turned out to be a pretty poor typist but it had been a good summer.

* * *

As the radiation progressed at Shands, Taylor turned once again to a source of comfort for her: poetry.

Taylor's Diary
March 11, 2001

Confusion.

Chaos.

That is all she can decipher.

No plan of attack.

No escape route.

A young woman stands shell shocked not knowing which
way to run.

The world around her proceeds normally. It is only
frightening to her.

And those she drags with her.

Once confronted by her demons all allies flee,

Unfamiliar with her burden they know not the real weight,

even the strongest of all is crushed by its massive size making

any hope of her relief somewhat impossible.

Chapter Twenty: Ebony and Ivory

Taylor was in ninth grade at Martin County High School and was home one day after school when I walked in from my own high school. I was surprised to see her doing her homework in the living room although, of course, the television was on in the background. I asked the all-too familiar question, but got an unusual answer:

"How was school today?"

"I stopped a fight." I remember she told me.

"Really? That was good. How did you do that?"

"Some black girls were about ready to beat up a white girl and I went over and stopped it. I went to Parker with the black kids and they knew me. All of the white kids who went to Parker get along with the black kids at high school, but the white kids who went to Palm City have problems with the black kids. How can anyone treat a person differently because of skin color? It's stupid."

It wasn't that Taylor was a civil rights leader. Obviously she was born after the Freedom Rides and the marches on Selma and Washington and she didn't know much of Martin Luther King's *I Have a Dream* speech save for the iconic phrase, but in a way in that moment, I realized for Taylor at least, Dr. King's dream had come true because Taylor was judging people on "the content of the character" not on the color of their skin.

All seven children in the family had attended J.D. Parker Elementary; it was certainly one thing which Pam and I agreed upon and all of the children had grown up with black friends in their lives. On the other hand, some of the kids who had gone to all-white elementary schools—some of Martin County's were 95% + white. Students who had sat at cafeteria tables together in first and second grade and shared peanut butter and jelly sandwiches and *Sip-ups* did not fight each other when they reached high school. They may or may not have been friends, but they had a common respect for one another. There were too many PB&Js, the sticky bonds of childhood, behind them.

I remember Taylor's comments were a revelation to me at the time. In the 1960s I had gone to Springfield High School in suburban Philadelphia and we had perhaps four black students attending the school, two boys and two girls. The Batipps brothers were great athletes so all of the white kids respected them, but I still heard comments in the hallways, an N-word here and there, words that too many folks still use. I had a good friend, Ron Dudley, who asked me if I wanted to invest in *Cloverlay*, a company set up to promote a young black fighter named Joe Frazier. The shares were $500 and I was afraid to risk my paper route money at the time for in the early sixties five hundred dollars was a tidy sum. So Ron bought two shares and after Smokin' Joe won the heavyweight title he cashed each share in for $32,000 I think. Ron and I went down to the Nixon Theater in Philadelphia to hear some Motown groups perform before the 1965 riots and we were the only white guys in the audience. There was never any trouble, never any fear, back then as there wasn't for Taylor.

Racism in America was far from dead, although I like to think it was terminally ill. But for Taylor and the black girls at Martin County High School that day, racism stopped for a moment, when the black girls, who were the ones acting like racists in this incident, were approached by a white girl who had been their friend since kindergarten. Kids, I realized, weren't inherently racist; they are raised that way. Red and yellow, black and white, they are precious in His sight. Somewhere along the line we forget what Jesus taught us, or Moses or Mohammad or Buddha if you prefer. In the words of Charley Pride, a black country singer: *We're all God's children, his next of kin…*

So, Taylor, the country hasn't come as far as you did, but perhaps someday it will.

Love, Dad.

* * *

Taylor's radiation treatment went on for several weeks with forays back to South Florida every other weekend.

Taylor's Diary
March 28, 2001

Well, I haven't been very adamant about writing everyday as you may have seen. Everything has been average up here in Gainesville. I found out today that I have to stay here until Apr. 16th. I am extremely anxious to go home. I mean, it's all right up here (much preferable to Durham) but I only have been home for two consecutive weeks in the last 4 months. And Dr. Friedman wants me to go 2 Duke for a consultation after I'm done here. I'm going to try to arrange for a week @ home before going up there.

Jeff and I are going strong although I get the distinct feeling that his family disapproves. But he has been incredibly sweet lately and he is an irreplaceable part of my support system. I don't know exactly where we go from here. But I am definitely dreading my prison time in Durham

107

because I know it will be upon me soon enough. Gia & Karly got an apartment & when I get there in Aug. I'll have to share a room w/Karly until Jan. I just keep looking forward to a time when the imperative thing on my mind will be studying for a mid-term.

Chapter Twenty-One: Katie Couric's Sister

I have never met the newswoman, Katie Couric, and she certainly wouldn't know me from Adam, but as I sat here reading *ACS College Scholarship Winner Enrolls in Life 101* with Taylor's graduation picture smiling out at me, I was reminded of two small coincidences that involved Katie Couric.

On September 11, 2001 when we were attacked by Osama Bin Laden, Sara Wilcox, the Martin County Superintendent of Schools, sent out an edict that all television sets were to be turned off. Coverage of the attack would cease. My country was under attack and Wilcox cut the cable connection. To say that she was a twit, is to insult twits. If she had been around on December 7th, 1941 she probably would have pulled the plug on Pearl Harbor reports on the radio if it hadn't been a Sunday and there was no school.

My high school kids couldn't find out what was going on. The next day I wrote a complaining letter to the *Stuart News* and within a week Sara Wilcox was talking to Katie Couric on *The Today Show,* trying to explain why she cut the cable to high school students during 9/11. Sara didn't do too well as I recall, from watching a videotape which was the South Fork High School equivalent of *America's Funniest Videos.* Poor Sara had been sandbagged by the cable-cutting question and had the look of a Ph.D. caught in the headlights of reality and prattled on about high school homecoming or some other banality. Taylor, at UCF, called me after the broadcast to say that Katie Couric quoted my letter to the editor.

"Did she mention my name?" I asked Taylor, my vanity aroused.

"No, Dad, she just said 'a teacher' and I knew it was you."

"How?"

"She used the word 'coddled' and I knew that could only be you. Who else used the word 'coddled,'" she teased.

True, I realized, I was just the type of teacher nerd to use an SAT vocabulary word anytime I could.

So it seems I had a part in making the school superintendent a fool in the eyes of the nation, and I was, at that moment, one of the strongest proponents for keeping teacher tenure, but as I reread the article about Taylor in the American Cancer Society newsletter, I recalled that in the same issue, the on-line magazine had mentioned the death of Katie Couric's sister.

There were pieces of the article about Taylor which sounded like conversations I had had with my daughter. How often had she told me a variant of:

Cancer changes you for the rest of your life. The little things don't bother you anymore and you get the beauty of every second that we have here. The importance of every day.

There were also portions of the article that would be phrases she would use at a speech at Disneyworld. *Mom, you're overreacting!* and *This can't be true. This happens to other people—not to me!*

And there were references of her going off to the University of Central Florida in spite of her brain cancer. I *didn't let my parents protect me too much. I didn't want to sit in bed; I wanted to do as much as I could. That was something I had to teach my folks.*

It was, I thought, she had to teach us that. And then there was the inference to boyfriend Jeff. She didn't think he would be the kind of guy to suffer through looking at a bald head and watching her throw up.

But that's the thing, Taylor said in the article. *People rise to the occasion and surprise you. And Jeff had replied, "whatever you're going through, I want to go through it with you." He even wants me to keep my bald head when my hair grows out.*

I had forgotten that about Jeff. Frankly I had forgotten the entire ACS article which is still on the internet (*ACS College Scholarship Winner Enrolls in Life 101*) and I had forgotten the coincidences with Katie Couric, who is now the anchor of CBS Evening News and still wouldn't know me from Adam.

Taylor's Diary
April 2, 2001

So I went home this weekend (from Gainesville). Karly & Charlie picked me up on Fr. afternoon. I got a ride home w/Otis's cousin Pearl (Otis was sister Beth's boyfriend and future husband). Her mom died of breast cancer when she was young. It was one of those situations where you meet someone by fate who brings something to light and then passes on through. She and I had a very enlightening conversation, and although I can't put a finger on what she gave me, it is definitely there. I spoke w/her about everything. It seems that every person w/whom I share this experience draws out a different aspect of the situation. So when I share different parts w/different people I am able to deal w/it and work through it piece by piece rather than sharing all of the overwhelming, indescribable emotions @ once. It's kind of like a dam, only a certain amount is dispersed @ at a time otherwise there would be a flash flood. Courtney, among others, seems to think that I don't talk much about how I feel about the situation, but what can you possibly say? It is beyond words. I have been so beat lately. I took a 6 ½ hr. nap today and I'm still tired. So w/that I bid you adieu.

Dad's Diary
April 4, 2001

I stood in for Taylor at Scholarship Night at Martin County High School since she returned to Gainesville this morning for radiation treatment. I even had my picture taken with the high school seniors as I "won" two scholarships.

I just wished Taylor could have been there tonight, but she was thrilled when I called her and told her the good news. To both of us, it is a sign of hope for the future.

Taylor's Diary
April 5, 2001

Last night I won 2 scholarships. Nina Haven which is $2000 yr/4 yrs. And Clementine Zacke Foundation for $2500/4yr. So, as you may have guessed I have a load off my mind now. Maybe now my life can start getting back on track hopefully.

Mom called today and said I have to do another round of chemo which I'm really against. Really, what is the purpose of suffering through that gagging when it didn't get past the blood brain barrier in the 1st place. Other than that my life is the same monotonous routine of doctors and hospitals. I'm so sick of everything. I am ready to get my life back again. I just kept thinking of everyone. I know Martin County starts Spring Break tomorrow and everyone is going to the Keys or Europe or somewhere. But where will I be on my Spring

Break of my senior year? Getting zapped in the head @ Shands Hospital. I can hardly contain my excitement. Today is just one of those days where the light @ the end of the tunnel seems miles and miles away.

A solitary tear slides down my cheek on its journey to the ocean,
Following a trail gallantly forged by its predecessors,
It keeps in constant motion, the night is dark and cold,
A coolness on my cheek, it numbs my whole insides
And begs me not to speak.
Gravity takes a toll and pulls with all its might
Yanks me from my hold into the day's sunlight.

Chapter Twenty-Two: Two Sisters

My little Florence Nightingale, a vision dressed in white
She comes when she hears my cries, and consoles me through
the night.
She tries so hard, to keep up that smile,
Unknowing I'm aware:
The walls are thin in this home, you see

And nothing is ever kept from me,
No drying tears or hiding fears.

I came across Taylor's poem about her sister Courtney the
other day and I remembered what Courtney had said to me
after Taylor's first brain surgery, as we walked hand in hand
along a hospital corridor.

"She's my best friend, Dad."

Not just a sister, but a best friend. And Courtney was
Taylor's nurse in a big way, having dropped out for a semester
at the University of Florida to drive Taylor to daily radiation
treatments at Shands Hospital. She also served as Taylor's
defender when CBS wanted to reschedule taping a radiation
treatment at Shands that would have delayed a visit home
past Good Friday. Like Taylor's favorite heroine, Katie Scarlett
O 'Hara drew strength from "Tara," Taylor drew strength
from home as well. Knowing how important home was to
Taylor's psyche, Courtney nixed the taping so the girls could
get to Stuart from Gainesville for Easter. She would later
protest to the CBS producers when they wanted to ask Taylor
certain questions. Courtney was Taylor's first line of defense.

So when Taylor had a chance to ask for a special occasion
from the *Make A Wish Foundation*—the wonderful organization

that takes sick kids to Disneyworld and other places—she chose something for Courtney.

I remember asking her why she chose a Stevie Nicks' concert.

"I did it for Courtney, Dad. Everyone always is doing things for me, but everybody seems to forget about Courtney. She's the one I've always counted on through all of this."

Not her mother, not her father, but Courtney. She was the one Taylor relied on: Her "Little Florence Nightingale."

"And *Make a Wish* will get us back stage so Courtney can meet the 'White Witch,'" Taylor added.

I asked her what she meant by "White Witch."

"That's Stevie Nicks' nickname," Taylor replied. She smiled at me. "You are really out of it, aren't you, Dad?"

"Uh huh."

"That's a good thing really," she added.

I think it was. If I knew too much about a group or a singer, Taylor would certainly think that performer was passé.

A limo picked up Taylor and Courtney and took them to a Stevie Nicks' concert in West Palm Beach and Courtney got a chance to meet her favorite singer backstage and Stevie chatted with the girls and gave them a drumhead from her band, a signed drumhead which became one of Courtney's prized possessions and is in her bedroom along with a lot of other things that she and her husband moved into my daughters' bedrooms for storage.

Sisters were truly something special I realized. There is so much emphasis on the bereaved parents when a child dies. *Compassionate Friends* is there for the parents, but sometimes people forget how devastating the loss of a sibling can be to remaining sisters or brothers. Taylor's death changed everything for Courtney. It changed her personality, her direction and her vision. It even changed the meaning of life for her. In spirit, Taylor has always been with Courtney, much more than she was with me. But then, they were sisters and best friends after all. And that bond was unbreakable even in death.

* * *

Nearing the end of her radiation treatment at Shands, Taylor made an entry into her diary. It was an exhausting time for her.

Taylor's Diary
April 11, 2001

Well, I went home this weekend and as usual it was very nice but very brief. I only have 3 more treatments left and I keep thinking how wonderful it will be this time next week. I will be @ home @ least for a brief respite. Dr. Friedman wants me to do chemo again but I'm not so sure about that because the last time we used a high dose and it didn't get past the blood brain barrier (rendering the chemo ineffective). So it was for nothing. What's to say that another kind would be any different? But, I guess we'll see about that.

So, Easter is this weekend and we're having a surprise baby shower for Kristine. I'm thinking about going to prom but I'm not sure. It's on the 21st of April. So it's in about a week. I don't know if that'll happen or not. If I do go I doubt Jeff will go w/me but who knows? Nothing really inspirational to say today. Maybe someday I'll become enlightened but for now my only realization is that I ought to sleep because I have a 10 o'clock appt. tomorrow. There are more important things in life than "things." I wish I could make my friends understand that. God never gives you more than you can handle.

P.S. On Mon. I slept for 18 straight hours. I have been dead tired.

Chapter Twenty-Three: You Betcha

I would never have thought a comment by Sarah Palin would stir my memory of Taylor's first driving lesson, but when the governor of Alaska said one of her catchphrase "You betchas," I suddenly remembered the first driving lesson I gave to Taylor. The mind is certainly a funny place.

Taylor was a few months short of her 16th birthday and she had her driver's permit in hand. It was the day to give Taylor her first lesson on the art of the stick shift and the driving of "Tammy Tercel," the 1991 car she so coveted. She referred to Tammy as "the Turtle" which I guess was okay since Taylor was the one who first dubbed the Tercel "Tammy." It is an idiosyncrasy of mine, passed down from my eccentric mother who drove "Bertha the Buick" and other alliterative autos over the years. So the kids had seen their father name "Daphne Dodge" and when "Daphne" finally clunked out, I went out and purchased a new Tercel. "Daphne" was so beat, however, they wouldn't even give me $50 on a trade-in. So I took "Daphne" home and promptly sold her for $200 to a Freddy- Fix-It type who kept "Daphne" on the road for another two years. Where was the "Cash for Clunkers" program when I needed it?

I remember my first chance to drive a stick shift on the hill of Locust Lane in Springfield, PA. My older brother Tom stopped his VW bug (the old-fashioned kind without the fuel gauge but with the emergency gas tank) on the hill, put on the parking brake, and told me to switch seats. So we rolled back to the bottom of the hill a few times, but then I got the feel of the clutch and we were off. The problem for Taylor, I thought, was an absence of spiffy hills on which to practice holding the car in place while getting the "feel" of the clutch.

At the time, Taylor had, on occasion, taken her mom's car out for a joy ride or two. It was a rite of passage among Pam's kids, drive mom's car before you actually had a license. So Taylor was familiar with the steering, but not the stick shift.

Years before I had taught my oldest step-daughter Tracey how do drive a stick shift and Tracey, the girls' big sister and surrogate mother, had wound up teaching the *H* pattern to the twins and Courtney, but Tracey was off living her life in Richmond, Virginia, and the job had reverted to me once again.

"Let the clutch out slowly," I advised Taylor.

Kerplunkkkkk! Kerplunkkkkk! The car stalled.

"More ah slowly," I suggested.

"Sorry, Dad," she replied.

"Try it again."

She turned the ignition, giving it the eerie screech. Then it was, Kerplunkkkkk! Kerplunkkkkk!

"Slower, Taylor, slower!"

"I'm trying, Dad. I'm trying."

"Did I ever tell you how Uncle Tom taught me the stick shift?"

"A million times, Dad."

"Oh."

"I think I'm getting it, Dad," she said. "It's a feel isn't it?"

"Yes!"

Magic does happen. Taylor let the clutch out slowly. The car didn't jerk, it moved smoothly.

In first gear.

"Now what?" Taylor asked me, a bit bewildered.

"Second gear," I replied. "Time to learn the gear pattern, just say *H*. It's an *H* pattern."

Second gear was not as difficult as first gear and after a bit of gear grinding she discovered second and we stayed in second gear and a solid 15 miles per hour as she drove us around the neighborhood. Linus might have his security blanket but Taylor had second gear. I was pleased with myself that I hadn't sworn once, and Taylor successfully returned the car to the driveway, a smile of satisfaction on her face and not even a scratch on the chrome.

"You're a good teacher, Dad," she told me.

"I had a great student," I replied, joining the mutual admiration society which Taylor had started.

"We are a great team, aren't we Dad?"

"You betcha, kid. You betcha."

Maybe I can tell her now what I didn't tell her then: she picked up the concept of the clutch much quicker than I had back on Locust Lane, but I suppose she knows that now.

You betcha I do, Pops. You betcha!

Chapter Twenty-Four: Writer's Block

We were on the Pediatric Oncology floor at St. Mary's in West Palm Beach and Taylor, between vomit-visits to the bathroom, was talking about what chemotherapy had taught her.

"You know, Dad. I don't keep my diary in the hospital," she said.

I asked why she didn't, and she replied and would later write in her journal:

I don't really write in here through chemo because I think of it like this: the time before and after the hospital is training for the match and then being in the hospital is like being in the ring, so you've got to go for the K.O.

I remember thinking that was an interesting analogy, especially for a daughter. I had no idea she even knew a thing about boxing for we had certainly never watched the sport together. I remember thinking Taylor looked like a boxer then. She was juiced up on steroids as prevention against a brain seizure or a stroke. But the steroids made her face puffy, like someone who might have been in a ring and been hit a few times.

"You know, Dad," she said. "Sometimes I just don't feel original. Why can't I write anymore?"

My aspiring poet had "writer's block"? I wondered if she really had writer's block. And then she showed me a poem in progress and I realized she could still write, at least in couplet form, her comfort food of rhyme. She would later add the poem to her diary.

I can't put into words my situation now,
It disappears somehow.
What are the emotions I'm supposed to feel,
Which is the method that will help me to deal
What do I need to gain in this lesson
And how will I know: do I just keep on guessing?
When all's said and done will I have gained what I should
Will I have learned all I could
About people and love, the purpose of living.
How will I know if I've gotten it right?
How I can I tell if I fought the good fight?
Where can I find what I'm to take from all this
Will I know right away or is it a hit or a miss?
I guess I will have to wait to the end
And discover whatever I've gained from it then.

When I finished reading the poem, I can remember my eyes tearing up.

"Is it that bad, Dad?" Taylor asked, startled by my reaction to her poem.

"No, no, Taylor. Don't worry, you can still write," I said.

"Well thank God for that anyway," she said and rolled her IV stand to the bathroom to vomit once again. "I don't know what I would do without my poetry."

* * *

April 22, 2001 was a tragic day for Taylor and Karly as their friend Justin overdosed on OxyContin and cocaine. A wealthy boy from Sailfish Point. He was dead at 19. "He can't be dead," Taylor cried when she heard the news. "He was on probation, he wouldn't do this." But the tears on her face

124

belied her words. She didn't write about it for two days and then only briefly.

Taylor's Diary
April 24, 2001

JUSTIN IS DEAD! He died 2 months to the day before his 19th birthday. I can't think straight. It doesn't seem real! These past two days have been one big haze. I don't even know how to grasp it.

Taylor's Diary
April 29, 2001

Well, the week from hell is finally coming to an end. I can't believe Justin is dead. I am so sad I can't even cry. He was such a big part of my life and now he's gone. I had to go to his viewing, that was so hard. When I walked up to his casket it felt like I was having a heart attack. I keep thinking that it can't be true. I mean it's Justin. Invincible diesel Justin. There was a thing @ the beach for him that was really nice. Then on Friday his funeral was @ St. Joe's. I didn't go to his burial but I got home from his funeral and just started writing a 5 pg. letter to him saying goodbye. So, later that afternoon I went and put it on his grave and stayed w/him awhile. I keep thinking that he's gonna wake me up in the middle of the night w/one of his infamous calls. And then he'll tell me that it was all some misunderstanding, that it wasn't really him lying in the coffin and then I'll bitch @ him for me making me so sad. Every night I hope he calls.

Chapter Twenty-Five: When the Bluebirds Sang

A week after Taylor died Justin Endicott's mother sent me a note that Taylor had written to her at her son's funeral the spring before.

> *Dear Mr. and Mrs. Endicott,*
>
> *I was compelled to write this poem about Justin because to me he was the bluebird of happiness. I am truly heartbroken about the loss of such a unique person. He impacted my life enormously and I have never, and definitely will never, meet another soul like him. I am sorry for your loss and for the loss for all the people that he impacted. He was an amazing person and he taught me so many things about life. I find comfort in knowing that a true angel is watching over me now. Sincerely Taylor Black*
>
> *P.S. I put the poem underneath his hand. I hope he likes it."*

And there was the poem in her typical couplet rhyme style:

> *Once I heard a bluebird singing in the night*
> *Undaunted by the darkness, without a trace of fright.*
> *He was unlike the rest, who slumbered why he played,*
> *Alone in the midnight, an enchanting song he made.*
> *I listened while he told me, things that struck me deep,*
> *I watched him as he danced while the whole*
> *World was asleep.*
> *But then as dawn was breaking slowly into day*
> *I gazed with my heart as my bluebird flew away.*

So, like any proud parent, I kept Taylor's poem after Mrs. Endicott sent it to me. Justin's death had really ripped Taylor up, the spring before she died. Taylor was sitting in the Lazy-Boy when Karly called with the shocking news. She began to cry and hyperventilate. Her knees were rubber and she couldn't stand up from the chair without my assistance due to the shock of learning of Justin's death. I was able to get her up and hug her, hold her close as she sobbed for her lost "bluebird."

I had shown Taylor a photocopy of my poem which I gave to Mrs. Freimuth when Bobby died and Mrs. Freimuth had it printed and passed it out at his funeral. The spring day after Bobby died, I slipped my hand-written poem into the Freimuth's copy of their *Philadelphia Bulletin*, for I was the neighborhood paperboy and in those days I put the paper inside the storm door so it wouldn't get wet. Looking back now, perhaps I gave Taylor the idea to write her own poem to Justin. I noticed I suffered from couplet-itis when I was a young writer as well.

A Friend of Mine
Gone is he, a friend of mine
One who was so true and fine;
To new horizons, he must go,
And leave his cheerful laugh behind,
The frontier unexplored is so,
He must explore and find,
The trueness of the Divine.
Gone is he, a friend of mine
One who was so true and fine;
No more will I hear him say,
Little wits as was his way.
Death has given him one last ride

To his Lord he will abide.
Departed, he, a friend of mine,
On one rainy April morn.
A guy named Bob who had been born
Some 16 years before his death.
A nicer boy I know not now.
Jesus spoke of greater fame-
'Death,' said He, 'Is an aim,'
For true life in the kingdom divine
Death then is a friend of mine."

I never wrote another poem that I can recall, except some substitute lyrics for songs like a Weird Al wannabe, but my mother kept that among her keepsakes and I found the original when we were going through her things when she died in January, 2003.

So Taylor, when I came across that old poem of mine written in, I believe, the spring of 1963 I didn't see Bobby Freimuth, I saw you, writing your poem to Justin and slipping it under his hand at the viewing. I saw you alone, visiting his grave in the weeks after the funeral.

Of course I never thought when I wrote that poem back in 1963 that I would ever have a child or lose a child to cancer like Mrs. Freimuth did, but perhaps if God's world had no time, my soul knew back then and I wrote the poem to comfort a future me as much as give comfort to Mrs. Freimuth. Bobby Freimuth, my *Monopoly* buddy who would shake the dice and say, "I'm barking for free parking" as he rolled the "bones" across the board. Somehow the past was connected to my future, and Taylor was another Bobby. That was certainly what Taylor might have believed. The karma of it all.

Taylor's Diary
May 5, 2001

I think about Justin everyday and I don't know how to handle it. I don't want to think about the fact that I have cancer. But I think I need to think about both of those things. I met Todd's friend Dave tonight. He worked at Sailfish Point and started talking about Justin as a boy. Both of his parents have been diagnosed with cancer and both are in remission and he knew Justin. There are no such things as coincidences! I ended up talking w/him for more than 2 hrs. I guess cause I've been avoiding everything God was sending a message saying, "look, here's a lesson you need to grasp." So I think I need to dig into that some more. I just hope I don't unravel.

Chapter Twenty-Six: All Dogs *Don't* Go to Heaven

Taylor always had an ambivalent relationship with Rhett Butler Black, a black dachshund who, at the time of his initial "kidnapping," was six years old. For the first six years of Rhett's existence he had been a bane to Taylor, and a blessing to Courtney, who was the family's dog lover. To Courtney, Rhett could do no wrong or so it seemed. Rhett was an irksome mutt to Chad because Rhett, not liking Taylor's brother, had once climbed up into the open cab of Chad's truck and left his calling cards on the driver's seat, both the number one and the number two "cards."

I certainly had no luck with dogs. I took Courtney's previous dog Gretchen out for a walk one night and she died on me, keeled over and croaked. Bad heart it seemed. I returned to the house with a dead pooch in my arms and from that time on I became rather fatalistic about animals in my life. But Rhett, like the girls, went back and forth between two houses and, on occasion when Pam's neighbors complained of Rhett's barking, Courtney would bring him to sanctuary at my house. But Rhett and Taylor never seemed to hit it off and Rhett, on more than one occasion, had left his calling card in Taylor's room.

The girls had named the dog after the fictional blockade runner from Charleston in *Gone With the Wind* although our Rhett yapped as much as Charles Hamilton, I thought. But what child would ever name a dog "Charles Hamilton." I mean the wimpy guy died of measles for heaven's sake!

Rhett's only saving grace, as far as I was concerned, was his penchant for climbing the rubber tree in the backyard. I thought he must be half-cat for he was as sure footed as a feline.

But one day after watching *The Princess Bride*, Taylor got the idea of kidnapping her sister's dog. In the film a "rodent of unusual size" or R.O.U.S was mentioned, and the ugly giant rat reminded Taylor of Rhett. So one day after school Taylor got home before Courtney and emailed her the following ransom note:

Courtney,

So you thought you could escape me? NEVER!!!!!!!!!!!!!

I have your little Rooskie Doodles (which was one of Courtney's nicknames for Rhett). Yip yip yip! That's him now. He hasn't taken much of a liking to his muzzle and little doggie chains that hold him as I allow rabid squirrels to dance in front of his cage, taunting him without end. Well, by now, you know the drill. I DEMAND $100 BAZILLION or I always wanted to know how weinersnitzel (sic) soup tasted and the old man (Dad) here is fattening up your precious little doodlebug every day. So if you ever want to see the little rat again I expect my $ in the next 24 hours. I think that is only fitting that as I write this, The Princess Bride is playing in the background- a sure sign that R.O.U.S. has only a short time left.

HAHAHAHAHAHAHAHAHAHAHAHAHAHAHAH AHAHAHAHAHAHA!

Signed

Xxxxxxx

Over the years Taylor repeated the kidnapping of Rhett, grabbing the dog and her bike and cycling to the other parent's house to drop the dog off.

I admit I was complicit in the kidnapping of Rhett and encouraging Taylor's mischievous creativity. She put a great deal of love into a practical joke, I thought, and sometimes now I envision her playing practical jokes in heaven, putting one over on St. Peter perhaps.

Later, after Taylor died, my sister-in-law visited Cassadaga, the Psychic Capital of the World in Central Florida, and informed me that Taylor was on the other side helping young souls in the transition from life to death. Like her mother who was an M.S.W., Taylor dreamed of being a social worker and, I like to think, perhaps she was now a "Soul-cial" worker. I don't dismiss anything anymore. I have had God work in my life and, I truly believe in angels. They may even walk among us. Or fly if you prefer.

Rhett died a few years after Taylor, but the movie title *All Dogs Go to Heaven* was made before Rhett came along, and if the movie makers had known Rhett they probably would have changed the title to *Most Dogs Go to Heaven*. Somehow I think Rhett might be yapping his lungs out in the Other Place, for he was a hell of a dog.

* * *

Although Taylor went to public school, she was a member of St. Joseph's Catholic Church and one day she was asked to speak to the parochial school's 8th graders about what she had gone through and how her faith had sustained her.

Taylor's Diary
May 9, 2001

I spoke at St. Joe's Middle School on Monday morning. That was the earliest I've been up in 6 months. There were 2 classes of 8th graders. I thought I was going to have trouble talking about it but it turned out surprisingly well. (Karly came w/me but didn't say a word of course.) Then later I spent practically all day getting an MRI. I got the results of the spine back yesterday and they were clear (no sign of cancer spreading). But I don't get the results of the brain back until tomorrow.

Let's cross our fingers! It's only 2 weeks until graduation on the 24th. I can't believe how fast it's gone by and I'll be going to college in the fall (at least hopefully if everything goes right). I feel like I've come to a block in coping w/Justin's death. I'm now @ the stage where it doesn't seem real and every time I think about it. I quickly change my thoughts. I just don't know how to cope w/a thing like this.

Justin has been such an important part of my life. He taught me many things and he definitely had a big impact on the person I've become. I just don't understand why he had to have such a short life.

Of course as Taylor's father when I reread that diary entry I just substituted the pronoun "she" for "he" in the last sentence of her entry.

Chapter Twenty-Seven: Drumsticks and Brain Tumors

Until one summer vacation when we made an ill-fated short cut across the National Mall in Washington to get from the Air and Space Museum to Natural History, Courtney and Taylor were carnivores. Unfortunately, Courtney was accosted by the PETA guilt-Gestapo. The PETA people showed her a number of ghastly images that were foul as well as fowl, and from that day on Courtney has not eaten a piece of chicken. She still eats seafood, but if it lives on land, she doesn't eat it. Thanks a lot, PETA.

Taylor, however, was made of sterner stuff or was, perhaps, indifferent to a drumstick's background or its family members, and during her treatment for brain cancer and her resultant use of steroids, Taylor developed a healthy appetite, especially for *Colonel Sander's Kentucky Fried Chicken*. And since the local KFC had an all-you-can-eat buffet I was able to keep Taylor in both cholesterol and calories without breaking the "Bank of Dad."

Ah, the smell of the plastic chairs and the gloss of the cheesy Formica tables which was the ambiance of the Colonel's grease pit, but Taylor and I didn't go for the atmosphere, we went for the feed, the mouthfuls of mashed potatoes smothered in the to-die-for chicken gravy, the coleslaw with the pleasing aftertaste and, of course, the secret recipe.

But we also talked.

"It's good to see you and Mom talking, Dad," Taylor said during one visit to the Colonel's restaurant. "Of course it took a brain tumor to do it."

I nearly swallowed a chicken bone when she made that comment, but it was an honest statement. I think, had Taylor not developed a brain tumor, I might have gone the rest of my natural life without ever speaking to my ex-wife. I envisioned myself as a Cal Ripkin of ex-husbands with over 2500 consecutive days without speaking to my ex-wife, but Taylor's illness had forced me to talk with Pam and work with her for the sake of Taylor; and my streak of silence was snapped and I failed to make it into the ex-husband's Hall of Fame. What neither Pam nor I truly appreciated was how painful it was for Taylor to be caught in the middle between two people she loved, who no longer loved but rather, loathed one another. Both Pam and I had forgotten the fact that there was once love, a love that was represented in the child before me, woofing down a spoonful of mashed potatoes. Many divorced parents, I believe, made that same mistake we did: forgetting they were once madly in love with an ex-spouse. I was sorry for that now, but of course it was too late. Yet that day I recovered from nearly choking on the chicken bone and replied to my daughter, "That's true, Taylor."

"I'm glad you are communicating. I need you both," she said. "I really do, Dad," she repeated for emphasis.

I looked at her and smiled, but didn't speak. She sensed I was uncomfortable talking about my relationship or, lack thereof, with her mother and conveniently changed the subject, "pulled a Nana," a tactic I had used so often when she was little, one that we had all learned from my mother.

136

"The steroids make me so hungry, Dad," she smiled. "You know, most people don't ever have anyone ever touch their brain during their lifetime and I have had people touching my brain in two different operations."

By that time Taylor had had the first brain operation at Martin Memorial Hospital North and, when the tumor returned, she had a second brain surgery at Duke University, performed by Alan Friedman.

"Sometimes I will step on something and feel it in my left foot and my right arm as well. It's like the wiring is off from people playing around in there," she said. "It's really weird sometimes, Dad. I don't think the brain is supposed to be played with like mine has."

I agreed with her. It didn't seem to me that God intended for people to mess around with brains as it was His territory, the seat of the soul. It should have been off limits. Taylor thought it all through very systematically, and came to the conclusion that the brain wasn't intended to be a toy, it wasn't something to be played around with, but then she really had no choice.

Taylor was overly fond of drumsticks and although I have eaten some KFC chicken in the years since, I have purposely avoided drumsticks. For several years I didn't eat a baked potato either. I guess I associated those foods with Taylor, but I had a baked potato not too long ago. However, I still haven't managed the courage to eat a KFC drumstick. Our favorite KFC franchise closed about two years ago and I like to think that without our business it went belly up. The booth we sat in so often to "pig out" during her steroid days may be long gone, but it was still fresh in my mind and I can see Taylor across the Formica tabletop, gnawing on a drumstick and talking about her brain tumor, a bit of the secret recipe juice squirting from the dead chicken's limb as she smiled at me. And she was with me once again.

My brain never was the same, Pops. It was if I had a short circuit or something, as if all the nerves had been crossed somehow.

You never let it bother you that much.

What was I supposed to do? There was nothing I could do, Pops. My brain was different.

So were you, Taylor. So were you.

* * *

To say that Taylor, a teenage daughter, had issues with her mother was akin to saying the Pope is Catholic, but still Taylor, ever the sentimentalist, never forgot a birthday or a Mother's Day. Grudgingly, she even appreciated her.

Taylor's Diary
May 13, 2001

Today is Mother's Day. I got mom some flowers and a card even though she deserves much more than that. I had a dream about Justin the other night. I saw his face and then it vanished. Then, I was asking him questions about death and everything. It all seemed very real. I still haven't come to terms w/it yet. I don't think that will happen for quite some time. No news from Henry (Dr. Friedman at Duke- he wanted everyone to call him "Henry.") but no news is good news as they say, right? Let's hope so. Mom and I both think he would've gotten back to us by now. Courtney just went back to Gainesville today. She's coming back on Fri. Kristine is supposed to have Anya any day now. I hope the munchkin

138

(niece Mikayla) won't be jealous. It's only 11 days until graduation. I can't believe it's gone by so fast. It doesn't seem like I'm old enough to be going to college.

Having cancer and going to college? Yes, in the spring of 2001 there was optimism for Taylor's condition. It seemed as if the radiation had worked and Taylor was put on a lighter chemo that didn't cause her as much nausea. Maybe, we thought, she could live a normal life after all.

Chapter Twenty-Eight: Giuseppe Zangara and the Homeless People

I often used Courtney and Taylor in the travel articles I wrote for magazines and newspapers. There was a two-fold reason for using the kids: 1) they were cute and people liked to read about cute little children saying the darndest things (Art Linkletter made a career out of eliciting such remarks), and 2) if I included them in the article in either a photo or in the copy, then I could deduct the money I spent on them as a business expense, which is why every summer when we went to Pennsylvania I wrangled a travel article for a Florida magazine or newspaper providing the periodicals stories about Longview Gardens, Pearl Buck's Home, the Kutztown Amish Fair or Sesame Place north of Philadelphia. I shamelessly used my progeny in a photo spread of the presidential homes of Virginia, having them pose at both Monroe's home and Jefferson's Monticello.

But one time Taylor and Courtney were with me when I had to drive to Miami to talk to the editor of *South Florida Magazine* for a couple of assignments to supplement my teacher's salary, and I decided to give my daughters a little history lesson and knock out a short history piece for the magazine to cover my expenses for the day.

In February 1933, Giuseppe Zangara attempted to assassinate president-elect Franklin Roosevelt at Bayfront Park in Miami (they inaugurated the president in March until 1937 when an amendment to the Constitution changed the inauguration date for the president to January of the year following the election). Imagine the world without FDR: whose profile would be on the dime? Reagan? Some

Republicans wanted to replace FDR on the dime with the Gipper, but the idea didn't fly. I say give Dutch the twenty-dollar bill and get rid of the Andy Jackson, who sent the Indians on the Trail of Tears. But that's another story.

In 1933 Florida's gun laws were as lax as they are today—heck, Florida is even geographically shaped like a pistol—and Zangara was a bipolar—or possibly schizophrenic—Italian-American immigrant who blamed kings and presidents for his ulcerous stomach. He might have taken a train to Washington and shot Herbert Hoover, the lame duck president, and people might not have cared that much, but Zangara read in the *Miami Herald* that the president-elect was in Miami on vacation and, what the heck, one dead president was as good as another for his sickly stomach, and it was balmy in South Florida, so why freeze his keister off in the cold of Washington D.C.? He might have been schizophrenic or bipolar, but he wasn't crazy. So he walked into a gun shop and bought a revolver and made his way to Bayfront Park one night to assassinate FDR. Unfortunately, he arrived a bit late and there was quite a crowd. Complicating matters, Zangara was vertically-challenged, being only a tad over five feet tall. So, to see over the crowd and get a good vantage point for a pistol shot, he had to grab a folding chair and stand on it. But still he couldn't see the president-elect clearly as FDR was sitting atop the back of a Buick convertible. Zangara, his stomach gnawing at him, fired the gun anyway and missed FDR by a number of feet, fatally wounding Anton Cermak, the mayor of Chicago. In response, the crowd ripped off some of Zangara's clothes and the cops came and took him away, a semi-naked, vertically challenged would be presidential assassin. Two months later,

Zangara would go to the electric chair for the murder of the Chicago mayor; some things *were* faster back then. When strapped to Old Sparky—the Florida electric chair—Zangara was asked if he had any last words and he replied with brevity, "Push the button."

But that early morning with my daughters, I wanted to find the exact location of the attempted assassination of FDR, and Taylor and we went to Bayfront Park, looking for the site. I was going to give her a history lesson after all, for that's what I was: a history teacher, when I wasn't moonlighting as a Hemingway-wannabe.

I found a plaque which stated that a hundred yards or so from that spot was the location of the failed assassination attempt of FDR. I pointed to the plaque for Taylor, but she pointed elsewhere.

"Daddy," Taylor said. "Who are the people?"

She was referring to a number of men who were sleeping on the ground in the park. It was a favorite spot of the homeless then, for the homeless often migrated south like the birds for the winter. Why sleep on a sidewalk grating in New York when you could sleep on the grass in Miami? Zangara would certainly have understood that.

"They are homeless men," I said, holding her hand and Courtney's as I navigated a path through the sleeping homeless.

"Why don't they go home?" she asked.

"Because they don't have a home, Taylor," I replied.

"That's sad," Taylor observed. "Can't we help them?" Her little face looked at me for an answer.

I could honestly say we couldn't, but Taylor was disappointed I couldn't do anything. After all, I was her father, her hero. Daddies were supposed to do everything. A tear of empathy rolled down her face.

We found the spot, but I was struck by the irony. It was at that park that Giuseppe Zangara tried to assassinate the man who started the New Deal, who put the homeless to work, and here in the park where FDR had nearly been murdered were homeless men lying all over the ground. I wondered what FDR would have thought. Taylor didn't understand the irony, she was too young, and she could only talk about the homeless men.

Maybe that was when Taylor decided to become a social worker and a knee-jerk liberal, or when the "progressive" seed was planted. Later, she wouldn't even remember the FDR connection to the park, but she never forgot the homeless men.

* * *

The day before Taylor was scheduled to graduate from high school, sister-in-law Kristine delivered her second daughter; Anya Taylor Pickard was named for her Aunt Taylor. "They named her after me, because I have cancer," Taylor said, although family members assured her that wasn't true which, of course, was a lie and she knew it. She was also chosen to be Godmother along with Beth. Beth was a backup she realized, "In case I die," she explained to me.

Taylor's Diary
May 23, 2001

This morning @ 9:24 Anya Taylor Pickard entered the world. She is absolutely the most precious thing ever. I can't believe it. She's such a mellow baby, too! Mikayla didn't really know what to think of her. In other news, I graduate tomorrow. I can't believe that's it. I'm done! I wish Katie could have been here for it. Afterwards, I'm going to Project Graduation. Everyone's coming tomorrow and we're gonna have a late lunch.

Oh, Jeff flipped his truck over. Some guy cut him off and he flipped. He's okay though. THANK GOD! Although he is on a few painkillers. It's been a month now since Justin. It seems like you go through life w/a normal set of problems and you think "ok" this sucks, but I can deal w/it. And then one day BOOM! The shit really starts hitting the fan. And you realize it was not so bad before. Then, after a year of constant bombardment of catastrophic situations overwhelms you, you search for the end of the storm, but there's not one in sight.

Chapter Twenty-Nine: Of Booth and Bill

A month after Taylor died, teacher colleague Martin Bielicki sent me a blown up photograph of Taylor on her eighth grade spring break class trip to Washington, standing outside Ford's Theater, wearing a *Gap Classic* sweatshirt and smiling through a mouthful of braces. Four thousand bucks as I recall.

It had been a coincidental moment as Mr. Bielicki and his wife had decided to take a spring break holiday as tourists in the nation's capital and ran into Taylor outside the theater where John Wilkes Booth shot Abraham Lincoln. Bielicki, a shutterbug, made a slide of the photo and the next year when Courtney was in his high school history class and he was presenting a slide show on the Civil War, he slid the Taylor photo into the mix, directing a question to Courtney who was totally surprised by the photo of Taylor outside of Ford's Theater.

When I see that photo today, I'm reminded of all the historical sites to which I dragged my daughters. Pam might take them to the Treasure Coast Square Mall, but it was my job, or so I thought, to take them to the National "Mall" and to a plethora of historical sites as well: Independence Hall, check. Pearl Buck's Home, check. Monticello, check. Mountain Vernon, check. Sagamore Hill, check. Gettysburg, check. Manassas, check. Brandywine, check. Ad nauseam , check.

* * *

When Taylor returned from the middle school trip she couldn't wait to tell me about it.

"I was the unofficial tour guide," she informed me. "I told everyone about Lincoln's assassination at Ford's Theater.

Showed them Booth's pistol. Even the teacher was amazed. I talked about Laura Keene and the play and how they stopped the play when the Lincolns arrived and about how famous Booth was and how he broke his leg when he dropped to the stage after shooting Mr. Lincoln. As in 'break a leg'."

"That's great, Taylor." I said

She beamed at my praise. It was at that point that I thought maybe dragging the girls to historical sites was beginning to pay off. Taylor went on. There was no stopping her. She was the star of the trip.

"And the White House was a blast again and so was the Holocaust museum. My teacher couldn't believe I had been to all of those places, Dad."

Boy, I was proud of myself as a father and a teacher, remembering how I had to schmooze my way into the Holocaust Museum by giving them my card with my "contributing writer" affiliation to South Florida Magazine. Pulling the press card was the only way to get in to the newly opened attraction—and fulfill a promise to Courtney. It was the same way I finagled a private tour of the White House for the girls and a photo of myself at the presidential podium in the press room, with the girls on either side of me, which I had made into a Christmas card, Taylor's favorite.

The White House press room photo also reminded me of a somber visit to The Wall, the Vietnam Memorial and a few moments with the engraved name "William G. Chandler" (1W62, August 11, 1972). I told Taylor the story of Bill Chandler. In elementary school we called ourselves the Mavericks; I was Bart to Bill's Bret after the popular western starring James Garner. Along with Bobby Freimuth, Bill

TAYLOR AND TIM BLACK

Chandler was my best childhood friend, but when I went off to college, Bill joined the army, went through Officer Candidate School, married a gal and had two kids, and was sent to Vietnam where he was wounded in action as a platoon leader. He recuperated at Valley Forge Military Hospital as I recall, and I saw him there. I was still in college, but when I graduated I joined the U.S. Army Reserves as my best chance to avoid Vietnam and was sent to Fort Lewis, Washington for basic training and A.I.T. Bill was stationed at Fort Lewis at the time, running a training company, and we reconnected. A couple of times he rescued me from the enlisted men's barracks to shoot pool and have a beer with him. He was a captain then and he didn't have to go back to 'Nam because of his wound, but he said if he ever wanted to make "field grade" (major or higher) that he needed more combat experience, since he didn't have a college degree. So he returned to Vietnam and he hadn't been there a month when a Viet Cong mortar round ended his life.

So I decided to visit the wall with my daughters and we looked through the large telephone book of killed-in-action for his name's location and I found his name and the location on the wall. There were the customary flowers and mementos at the base of the wall, notes inscribed to the ghosts of another time, a war growing more distant every year. Photos of the deceased. In uniform. As children. A teddy bear from a child I guess. Or maybe it was the soldier's as a little boy and his mother left it for him. The sorrow was palatable

And then we found Bill, at my eye level, but over my daughter's heads and I lifted them one at a time to see his name, to touch the engraved letters of a name that once had

149

meant so much to me. Then I set the girls down and began to cry. As I was with my children I thought of Bill's two daughters, fatherless, and how they were probably grown women now, perhaps with children of their own, and how Bill had missed so much in dying so young. He had not only missed his own life but his daughters' lives as well. I felt guilt for not keeping in touch with his widow, but then I only met her once, I believe, and darned if I could even remember her first name or where she moved after Bill was killed. She might have even remarried and changed her name.

But I remembered Bill; he was etched in my memory as deeply as the engraved letters were in the Wall, and my daughters seemed stunned that I was crying. Taylor looked at me with her big brown eyes and a tear empathically escaped down the side of her face.

"You miss your friend, Daddy?" she asked.

"I do," I said, giving her a hug.

She handed me a piece of tissue. I blew my nose and smiled at her.

She gave me a big hug and I was back from the dead and among the living once again.

Taylor's Diary
May 28, 2001

Well, I graduated! I can't believe I'm finished. This school year (or lack thereof) is one in which my life has changed forever. Nothing about this year has been calm or docile, rather it has been draining and perturbing and so many other multitudes of things. It is something that cannot be understood until you are in that situation. You encounter so many different feelings physically, emotionally and spiritually. Only others who have come before you and those who will follow will ever comprehend the epiphany that is cancer. This is just as cancer victims cannot grasp family and friends change of emotions. I do not know what I'm supposed to have learned from this, but I do know that it is the key to my soul's unrest. I have been so irritable and angry. I can't put my finger on the exact source. Instead, it seems to be many things. I suppose I'll just have to work through this. My life right now is full of uncertainty. And while everyone is enjoying their last summer @ home or taking summer classes, I will be imprisoned in a hospital room at Durham N.C.

Ah, such is life! And in the words of my father, "@ least you're alive." Oh, how true that is.

Perhaps I should have been more upbeat in my advice, but I was grateful that Taylor was still with us and wanted her to feel grateful as well. She had survived two brain operations, radiation and rounds of chemotherapy and on the day she graduated she seemed healthy.

Cancer though, is a rollercoaster. Sometimes a patient is up, other times she is down. The patient is in the front car, but the family is also on the ride with her from the heights of hope to the depths of despair. That night at graduation, I could hear Frank Sinatra singing *High Hopes* in my head.

Chapter Thirty: On the Beach

One evening on television the black and white film *On The Beach* was telecast with Gregory Peck wooing Ava Gardner "down under" in a post-apocalyptic world while, in the background, tipsy Aussies, oblivious to the increasing radiation levels, were singing *Waltzing Matilda*. As the world was ending on screen, my mind was taking me to another beach, Bathtub Beach on Hutchinson Island.

When my daughters were little I often took them to Bathtub Beach in Stuart, a beach which has been hammered by hurricanes and erosion, but was once the favorite family sandbox in the area. A natural reef formed a "bathtub" and little children could wade into the water while parents sat on the shore, unconcerned that their little ones would drown in water that didn't go over their heads at low tide. It was where Taylor met the ocean and fell in love with the sea. A half-mile off Bathtub Beach her ashes mixed with the current, so in a way Bathtub Beach was a beginning and an end. South of Bathtub Beach is the exclusive gated community of Sailfish Point, but even that beach is public up to the dune line.

Taylor and I walked onto Bathtub Beach one evening a few days before her eighteenth birthday for what would be our last walk together to the inlet at the end of Sailfish Point. It would be on such a walk that Courtney would meet her future husband Robby, and it was on such a walk with Courtney, Robby and Robby's parents that I thought of my last walk with Taylor on the beach as Courtney and Robby's little dog Camden scampered ahead in the sand.

During her cancer, Taylor often walked the beach for the serenity of it all. It was early January in 2001 and Taylor said it was the most beautiful day of the year thus far. We walked to the inlet and as she recorded in her diary:

The sun was shining brilliantly on the ocean, which was a thousand shades of blue and green. It was definitely one of God's most spectacular creations.

But even with the beauty we still had to discuss the upcoming stem cell "harvest" at Duke.

"I'm not looking forward to that, Dad," she said.

"I know, and you need another MRI."

I always thought she took the claustrophobic conditions of the MRI extremely well, but then Taylor had learned to accept things I don't think I could have ever accepted.

"You know, everything's been good lately, Pops. I am confident that I will beat this. It only wins if you let it win." It had become her mantra. I knew she was her own best cheerleader, and she said some things aloud to give herself confidence. But then, I do as well. I suspect a great many people do.

And then she spoke about Otis's mom doing some type of holistic healing that dealt with energy flow in one's body. She was optimistic that it was having some salutary effects. We weren't quite as desperate as the actor Steve McQueen had been, going to Mexico to take some promised wonder drug. There is always a charlatan ready to sell a desperate patient a cure for cancer; there always has been I think, but there was no cost involved in the treatment and it certainly could do no harm and might help her psyche at the very least.

"It is soothing and I have a feeling that it will have positive effects." Taylor said at the time.

154

I asked her about her friends. The last time she had been in the hospital the visits from her friends had dropped off and I made the mistake of saying something about it and it had made her cry, so I never mentioned it again. The novelty of a friend's illness wears off quickly for teenagers, I realized, and they slowly lessened their visits over time but when Taylor was out of the hospital she plugged into her network of peers. But she had written about it in her diary.

I haven't seen much of anyone lately. Everybody's into their boyfriends. Hopefully I'll hang out with them soon. Karly and Gia went to Orlando without me. I have a feeling they want to move in together, just the two of them. Life is so short and there is no use letting things like that get to you. You just got to let things go.

"I'm going to start doing meditation everyday at the beach, Dad," she said as we walked along the shore. "I had the most terrible dream about Jeff last night. It seemed so real, and I woke up and was uneasy for a couple hours."

She alluded to some type of a car crash, as I recall now, which, in retrospect may have been prescient, but who is to say? We then talked about her upcoming eighteenth birthday. She would be an adult in the eyes of the law.

"Looking back my life was very different and promises never to be the same," she said philosophically. "Well, Dad, you always said 'change is constant.'" Her smile was wistful.

A few weeks later the tumor would return and everything that was going well would go the other way, but that night on the beach we had a chance to walk and talk and I got a chance to see my daughter as a young woman and not as a little girl. It wasn't as scary as I had feared, as I suppose every father fears, when his daughter completes the journey from childhood into womanhood.

Taylor's Diary
June 6, 2001

There is an indescribable emotion that forever haunts people who have lost someone they love.

It is something that cannot be understood until someone has experienced it personally. Let me just say I wouldn't wish that hurt on anyone. And although they say time heals all wounds, this is the exception. This wound never healed. I went to Duke last week. It wasn't really good news, but it wasn't really bad news. I'm going to have to begin taking chemo pills awhile. They are 5 pills for 5 days out of the month. Supposedly these pills have very little side effects, if any. So maybe after months of baldness (and wigs) I can finally have some hair again. I'm extremely excited that this won't interfere with school @ least for a while. I am ready to begin a new chapter in my life. I have finished Ch. 1 "The Stuart Years." I'm going to take a summer class w/Karly now that the stem cell is postponed. I need to get back in the groove of things.

The visit to Duke showed there was still a residue of tumor so Taylor wasn't able to start the isolation and stem cell replacement which would have been end of the protocol. So, instead, the Duke doctors put her on a lighter form of chemo and told her to go off to college and live her life. Perhaps this should have been a harbinger, but we didn't realize it.

Chapter Thirty-One: A Last Drive Through Valley Forge

My mother's house in Wayne was located but a short drive from Valley Forge National Park, and on summer evenings I would chauffer my mother and my daughters over to the park to watch the deer romp across the pastures where once George Washington and his army had encamped through a terrible winter. I always thought that George would be surprised—and I hope pleased—that the fields on which his troops suffered were now populated in the summers by white collar workers on lunch breaks and couples canoodling beside their picnic blankets near the areas where the Revolutionary War soldiers nearly froze their breeches off.

Valley Forge was also a place where I took the girls for a bike ride, amused that they were winded by the small hills we pedaled up and down, for they had only ridden bicycles on the flat paths of Florida and, unlike northern kids, they were unaccustomed to inclines and didn't know how to conserve their energy.

It was at Valley Forge as well, that I taught my daughters the delicate art of skipping stones across streams, impressing them with my uncanny ability to uncork a "triple skipper." We would often stop by one meandering brook and toss our stones in the stream. The girls looked forward to this as a daily ritual when we were in town visiting Nana.

So on a trip with Taylor to see "Nana before she died" as Taylor requested, and what I really took to mean, *in case I die,* Taylor asked for a last ride through Valley Forge before we drove to the Philadelphia airport for our flight back to Florida.

For Taylor, Valley Forge was a sanctuary, a reminder of all that was good about her childhood, when there were no such things as ports in one's chest to deliver the chemotherapy, when hair was long and luxurious and every moment of summer vacation promised magic in the next breath, when the most important thing in the day was the possibility of a "triple skipper" across the stream with the covered wooden bridge.

I drove a back way into the park, up past the ceremonial arch, parking by the spring-fed water fountain that Taylor had always loved as a girl. The water was as cool and refreshing as it had always been, and Taylor stood beside the car, just looking away toward the soldier huts a few hundred yards in the distance.

"Do we have time to stop at the stream, Dad?" she asked.

I said that we had plenty of time. One of the side benefits of being a tad anal was that I was nearly always early for everything. While it was suggested a customer show up ninety minutes early for a flight, I might show up three hours before takeoff, so we had plenty of time to dawdle in the park before the flight.

I parked the rental car by the spot we had always parked, down the way from the covered bridge. The girls had always crossed a small pedestrian bridge which forded the stream but to our surprise, that bridge was no longer there.

"That's not right," Taylor said as we stood by the car, stunned that the pedestrian bridge was gone. "Things aren't supposed to change here. This is frigging Valley Forge. That isn't right, Dad."

It was cruel. It was if the forces of nature had not only given Taylor a brain tumor but had taken away a revered memory of childhood.

"How do the kids get to the other side of the stream to throw their skipping stones?" she asked me.

I didn't know, nor was I ready for her tears. Taylor began to cry. Cry for the lost pedestrian bridge, cry for the change of it all, cry for the broken memory of childhood, shattered like some porcelain doll by the awful hand of fate. Or maybe she was crying for herself and what she was going back to: the unknown future.

There at Valley Forge she had felt secure in the past until the present intervened and reminded her that change comes to all people and all things, even a national park.

We didn't stay long after that and I drove on to the airport and we returned to Florida.

Taylor's Diary
June 14, 2001

I write to you from my Nana's attic, one of the most comforting places in the world for me. I always thought, If there is one thing that is constant in this world it is my Nana's house in Wayne, P.A. I have come to the conclusion that there is nothing constant in this crazy world. I have not seen Nana in 3 years, up until now. She has aged a lot in that time. She has a sweet woman that lives with her now and helps her out. She still knows what's going on but sometimes she is a bit forgetful. Enough so that we have not told her about my disease. It would confuse and frighten her. Hell, it confuses and frightens me. So, needless to say I have spent the majority of my stay peaking around corners to see if I needed to put my wig back on before she saw me. But, it is a pilgrimage that I needed to take in light of the past year I've had I needed to find solace and retreat once more to my comfort zone. What I found here was change, which only reiterated the fact that I need to move forward and start anew. Having said that, our trip concludes on Sunday. And I leave for Orlando on Monday. I haven't even packed yet, although I really don't need to take anything but clothes just yet. I hope the girls can be convinced to break the lease early. Otherwise, I'll be feeling like a guest until I get my own bedroom. And so begins "Ch. 2! The Disney Years."

Chapter Thirty-Two: Oprah

One day Taylor introduced me to Oprah Winfrey and I became secretly addicted to the TV program *The Oprah Winfrey Show*. I suppose admitting my powerlessness about *Oprah* was a first step, but for years I was in denial; I was a man and I was watching *Oprah*. Except for my daughters, my secret remained buried in the closet. Like a great many addictions it began innocently enough: with experimentation.

Often after school at 4 p.m. Taylor would turn on the tube to the Empress of Empathy, pop some popcorn, and bring out the butter spray; it was the no-cal butter spray, the *I Can't Believe it's not Butter* spray in the yellow plastic bottle that she sprayed as liberally as the county trucks spraying for mosquitoes. Beside the popcorn bowl would be the ever present Diet Coke. One family member would later wonder if the soft drink contributed to Taylor's brain tumor, but we discounted that theory.

One day Taylor asked me to join her and a bonding was begun: I watched *The Oprah Winfrey Show* with my daughter, a box of tissue, strategically placed on the coffee table between us. One never knew when Oprah would tug at one's heartstrings with a segment about starving autistic disabled children from Appalachia who had become orphans due to a mine disaster in which their father died and their mother subsequently died a day later of grief associated with the loss of her husband. So a tissue box was always at the ready in our house.

As I said, *Oprah* addiction wasn't the type of thing that a man easily admitted, but the programs were fascinating and later when Taylor was undergoing chemotherapy at St. Mary's

Hospital, I would sit in the chair beside her hospital bed and click on *Oprah* for her and for myself. When her sisters were with her in the hospital they would watch *Oprah* with her as well. One hour of someone else's suffering could be strangely therapeutic to a young girl on chemotherapy. Look, just for today, someone else has it bad as well. Misery does indeed love company. Why do we rubberneck at highway accidents? Why do we slow down? Isn't a part of us saying, "there but for the grace of God go I"?

For Taylor the power of Oprah's program was truly remarkable. I rarely watch the program anymore; not that I've joined Oprah Anonymous or anything; my reason for watching the program wasn't Oprah, it was Taylor and sharing time with her. With Taylor gone, well, so was my desire and my reason to watch the Queen of Talk Shows.

In retrospect, the programs all seem to blend in my mind except the ones where Oprah gave away this or that. I don't believe Taylor was still alive when Tom Cruise did his famous couch hurdle, but for a couple of years we followed the issues and the dysfunction of many of the guests and even caught local attorney, Willie Gary, as he and his wife were introduced in Oprah's audience. Gee, I knew a guy who was on Oprah's show, I could say. Ironic I suppose that Willie Gary would also be featured on *60 Minutes* as well as Taylor. Funny too, that the three people from Stuart who had been featured on *60 Minutes* were people I knew. I even taught with Barbara Webb whose dentist injected her with the AIDS virus. Mrs. Webb made the "Stopwatch Show" as well.

Today *Oprah* is a short stop on an occasional remote control "channel surf." Oh, once in a while, the *Oprah* addiction will have its way, and I'll watch an entire episode, but missing is Taylor's call of, "Hey, Dad, *Oprah's* coming on." Watching *Oprah* is not the same without Taylor. Sometimes after a few minutes of *Oprah* a lump comes to my throat that I think Oprah's viewers would understand.

Taylor's Diary
June 19, 2001

Well, I'm here. Thank God! I'm here! (Taylor was in Orlando for a community college class before the fall semester at the University of Central Florida). I need to have a fresh start in a fresh place. Put last year behind me. The only thing I'm missing is Jeffery. I am really missing him. Over the past year he had been my rock. He has helped me sooooo much,

Well, I started the chemo pills on Sunday night and so far I've had very little nausea. But last night I had pains in my stomach. This chemo is called Temodar. It has 5 vials, each filled w/3 pills, 2 white ones and a brown one. It seems I have to do 4 rounds or so (Depending upon how it works). Supposedly, this kind is not going to make me lose my hair. But, really, I gotta see it to believe it!! You know what I mean? I'm beginning to think I'm never going to get any hair back. I've been hairless for a nearly a year now. And although the novelty has definitely worn off I will say that everyone must have a bald head once in their lifetime. It is certainly a unique experience and one which cannot be explained properly except to say that it must be experienced @ some time or another.

I started my class today. It's called Student Success. It's supposed to teach us time management and study skills, some things I need to learn. I'm debating whether or not I'm

163

going home this weekend. I want to see Jeff and I need to get a few more things to bring up here. But on the other hand I need to spend some time up here. I guess we'll just see what happens in the next few days.

Chapter Thirty-Three: Blame It on the Brain Tumor

Obviously there is nothing humorous about a brain tumor right? One would think so, but for Taylor the brain tumor did have some amusing benefits; it became her catchall excuse for her mistakes, and even her misbehavior, and besides, her friends liked to hear the sloshing and thumping sounds in her head. One time I caught a few of them in line waiting their turn to hear the inner workings of Taylor's noodle.

"Hey, Dad, want to hear my brain?" Taylor asked me after recovering from her first brain surgery. The surgeon had replaced the piece of skull he cut off to get to her brain, of course, but there was indeed a tell-tale slosh when she shook her noggin. "My friends think it's neat," she added. I could only listen to it once, and I was sorry I did. She could see the discomfort on my face and laughed at me.

"You shouldn't laugh at your father, Taylor," I said, though a thin smile gave me away.

So she laughed again.

Shortly thereafter, the brain tumor became a handy excuse for all of the dents on Tammy Tercel and the *D* in Geometry. Taylor was a regular Fraulein Fender-Bender with the broken back up lights and crumpled bumpers, and now she had the perfect excuse for her mini-accidents: the brain tumor. Certainly the brain tumor had a really big downside, but Taylor was an adolescent and one thing adolescents need as surely as air itself are excuses for their misbehavior. My dog ate my homework is obviously trite, but a brain tumor is a veritable gold mine for the excuse factory. A brain tumor evokes immediate sympathy: you poor thing, of course you back-ended me, what else could you do, you have a brain tumor. Pity, sympathy, all of these were possible upsides of a brain tumor. You poor thing, couldn't master Geometry. Why you don't know it yet, but you have a dormant brain tumor and someday it will give you the perfect angle you can use on your father to explain your deficiency in Geometry. It is too bad that Taylor didn't live back with Socrates and Plato, because she came up with a Brain Tumor Philosophy.

"A brain tumor has an upside, Dad," she informed me of her new epistemology. "It really gives me an excuse for a lot of things."

It was an odd way to look at things, but then, so is stoicism. Taylor did have a sense of the absurd. In Martin Memorial a week before she died when she was waiting for a bed in the local Hospice Residence, Aunt Barbara was in the room with her when suddenly Taylor asked to use Barbara's cellphone.

"Who you gonna call?" A surprised Barbara asked her.

And Taylor had brightened with a big smile as if fed a set up for a great punch line and replied, "Ghostbusters."

No, she didn't hum the theme to the movie, but there was a bit of irony in the comment as she had begun to see things in the hospital room that we couldn't see. Was it the morphine, or was it something else? Albert Einstein's last words were reported to be "now come the answers" and I suppose we only learn the answers when we check out of this place.

Now Taylor was not about to write "Brain Tumor the Musical," and there were certainly more days of rain than sunshine for her, but a laugh could lift her spirits and get her through the next day.

The doctors suggested that Taylor had the brain tumor at birth. I was in the delivery room with Pam, as I had been for Courtney, a great Lamaze Coach whom Pam basically dismissed during a series of contractions that brought Taylor forth into the world not through any assistance of her "coach."

The gas guy during the delivery made some waggish comment to me about being a "brute" to cause my wife's discomfort, but he atoned for his bad humor by getting little Taylor's lungs functioning correctly.

Was it there, I wonder now, right there in the delivery room, that Taylor had a brain tumor? The doctors' theory was the tumor lay dormant to late adolescence and with Taylor's changing body, it developed as well. If so, it might explain Taylor's childhood klutziness, her two broken arms.

Maybe she had the brain tumor from Day One and she was fated for a short life, maybe that's why she said when she was four and five years old that she wasn't going to be here long, and that at seven she said she saw heaven. Maybe we can truly blame it on the brain tumor after all.

Taylor's Diary
June 26, 2001

Well, I went up to Duke and had an MRI done. Also talked to 60 Minutes. The results were pretty much the same as last time. There is something there which leaves us on the same path as before. So, not much news there. I'm just going to continue w/the Temodar and see how that works. 60 Minutes was an experience. I was excited that I got to speak with Ed Bradley. He's so easygoing; he made me feel very comfortable spilling my life story on national television. Remind me to vacate the country when it airs.

In other news, not a whole heck of a lot. I am writing to you from the Raleigh/Durham Airport, patiently awaiting our flight home. I'm getting used to living on my own. I just desperately need my own bedroom because I feel like a guest. But, Gia and Karly are in their own little world and I think they like it just fine and dandy w/only the 2 of them there. You know what they say, "three's a crowd."

Chapter Thirty-Four: J. D. Salinger and *A Land Remembered*

I was reading on the internet that the reclusive author J. D. Salinger was suing another author for using his character Holden Caulfield from *The Catcher in the Rye* for some rip-off rendition called something like *Shortstop in the Wheat Germ* and Taylor came into my head once again:

I read all of his stuff, Pops, remember?

Yes.

I mean what book better captures adolescence than Catcher?

None that I can think of.

I don't know how many times I read that and Franny and Zooey.

Taylor discovered J. D. Salinger at roughly the time that she discovered boys, at say thirteen or fourteen. Like many teenagers who discovered a new author, she thought he had written especially for her, for if there was anything certain in the teenage universe it was that the teenager herself was the center of it. Kind of like Ptolemy's idea of the cosmos, with the earth as the center.

But I think the book that she and I most discussed was a saga of Florida history written by Patrick Smith: *A Land Remembered,* a novel set in Florida from before the Civil War through the 1960s, and the only book that the red neck kids at South Fork High School had ever read cover to cover. It was a captivating family saga with racial undertones as it didn't spare the language of the Florida "Cracker." It was in *A Land Remembered* that Taylor learned the origin of the moniker "cracker" for the cowboys who cracked their whips while herding cattle. She also learned a good deal more about Florida history than she had in her fourth grade class.

As a divorced dad with no money to spare, my girls and I spent endless evenings in the local library, and Taylor became a library addict. Books gave her the opportunity to escape to another time or place or to visit another person and, of course, nurtured her desire for poetry.

She was unusual among her peers, as was Courtney, for being such an avid reader. While Courtney was a full-fledged nerd, Taylor always had one foot in nerd-land and one foot in party-ville.

I gave you fits, didn't I, Pops?

Yes, you did, Taylor.

You don't know the half of it, she laughed. I was like you were when you were in college, Pops.

Yes, my undergraduate days at Gettysburg College at the Phi Delta Theta house. Not quite as bad as Belushi's *Animal House*, but bad nonetheless. I skirted by with grades which were just good enough to keep me from being drafted and joining Bill Chandler on the Wall in Washington. I wanted to put my Gettysburg past behind, so a few years after I graduated, I sent a phony letter to the class secretary, who had always been naïve in college, saying that I had died in a hang-gliding accident off the coast of California. I signed a buddy's name, of course, and after the next issue in which my death was reported I no longer received solicitations from the alumni clubs for cash. Of course, my mother was rather upset with me, but it was a small price to pay for a lifetime without solicitations from alma mater.

170

Our generation just did it a few years earlier than you did, Pops, Taylor used to say about her generation's misbehavior. What my generation did in college, hers did in high school and today's are doing even earlier.

Today, students begin experimenting with alcohol and drugs as early as middle school, some even in elementary school. On any given weekend more high school students are finishing a six-pack than are finishing a book, but I suppose Taylor did both.

Like many parents, I have learned things about my children after the fact. In Taylor's case, I learned a great deal after she died. I learned she was as flawed as any other human being. Normally, I think, we find out things about our children's adolescence when they are safely in their mid-twenties. I think I was 25 or 26 when I finally told my mother that Bill Chandler and I, playing with matches, had burned down a field when we were 13. Got away with it too.

So when I think that my children are not the objects of perfection that I had once envisioned, I try to remember myself as the incorrigible little miscreant I often was. Holden Caulfield would understand that about all of us.

Taylor's Diary
July 1, 2001

Well, I write to you from Orlando. I am sitting in my apartment watching "Goonies." Although it doesn't really feel like my apartment. I don't even have a bedroom. Supposedly, we are getting a 3 bedroom in August, but Gia and Karly each have a bedroom and they don't seem anxious to move. Jeff just left today. He came up for the weekend and we had a really nice time. I really didn't want him to leave.

171

He moves to N.C. on the 6th. We're gonna try the long distance thing and see how it works. I'm going to try so hard because I think we were meant to be. I mean he came into my life right before the shit hit the fan. I would have never thought that he of all people would have been able to be as understanding and caring as he has. He really has been my saving grace. Without a doubt. And if we have made it through the last year and he hasn't bailed on me he is definitely a long term keeper. I keep thinking about Justin. It doesn't seem real that he's dead!!! It can't be. I don't know how to deal w/that. I can face my own mortality but not his!

Chapter Thirty-Five: Dido and the Grandfathers

When I think of those horror movies like *Halloween* or *Nightmare on Elm Street* I recall that they all had sequels, in some cases, several sequels. So perhaps Taylor should have been prepared for *Brain Surgery II, the Sequel!*

You weren't ready for that setback, were you, Pops? She whispered to me the other day.

No, I certainly wasn't ready for that. A few days after her 18th birthday Taylor was at Pam's and throwing up, not from the chemotherapy but from something else. It is truly amazing when you hope your daughter merely has food poisoning, for in your mind you are thinking the dreaded tumor has returned, that ugly friggin' tumor, and that the damn chemo hasn't worked, that maybe she should have had radiation first. But there is no Monday morning quarterbacking in brain tumor treatment as far as I'm concerned. It really doesn't matter if you should have called a different play if the patient was dead. The end zone is literal. But this was still early in the "game."

So Taylor had an MRI at St. Mary's which indicated that the tumor had indeed returned. I was with Taylor, mulling over a decision as Pam had gone off to try to see Dr. Paul. Taylor and I couldn't reach Pam by phone. Taylor needed surgery. A kind-hearted nurse tried to help Taylor and me with the decision.

"What do you think, Dad?" Taylor asked me.

I turned to the nurse for advice.

"Our neurosurgeon is incompetent," the nurse said. "I wouldn't let him work on my dog."

I remember Taylor's eyes growing larger at the comment. Well, that was pretty damn honest, her face seemed to say. The problem was that it was the weekend and the pediatric oncology team wasn't around to discuss the needed surgery.

The nurse was gung-ho about Duke.

Then, as if clairvoyant, Henry Friedman from Duke called Taylor in the hospital. Duke's neurosurgeon, Alan Friedman, was "the Michael Jordan of brain surgery; he was the best in the world," Henry said. "Come to Duke, we'll take care of it." The phone call clinched Taylor's decision although we would have to wait until the following day for release from St. Mary's. Pam would make the trip with her.

"I trust Henry," was what Taylor said. I hadn't met Henry Friedman at that point, but I had researched his career and it was stellar. He was recognized as one of the best neuroncologists in the nation.

I was rereading Taylor's journal entry from January 18, 2001.

> Well it's amazing what can happen in one week. I am up at Duke but not for the stem cell harvest. Instead, I have come back for a second brain surgery. It all started two days after my birthday. I started to have severe headaches and vomiting. So I went down to St. Mary's to do an MRI, and they found out the tumor is back and bigger. So here I am, lying in a hospital bed at Duke and having arguably one of the worst evenings in my life thus far. It has taken them about five hours and four people and one thousand sticks later. Finally, I have it in and I'm extremely frustrated. I can't even decipher the array of emotions.

The following day she had surgery and at 4 p.m. I received a collect call from Taylor in ICU.

"It was really neat, Dad," she said about the surgery.

"Neat"—that's what she said, it was neat and in a way it was. I know it was "neat" she had come through surgery successfully. What a difference from the first brain surgery when Taylor had spent so much time sedated. I recorded Taylor on tape when she talked about her second brain tumor operation.

"It was surreal, Dad. First, they put me under and then they woke me up and there was a special doctor, Dr. Robbins, I don't know who he was. He was in charge of making sure I kept all my motor skills and brain functioning while Dr. Friedman—Alan, not Henry—was working on my head. So he had me doing simple motor skills with my left side and even with my right side—about an hour of lifting my leg and tapping my hand and saying the date and the year and things like that. That was probably about an hour. I could hear them debulking the tumor the whole entire time. It was kind of like the drill sound of a dentist that you hear. You could feel the sensation but it wasn't like pain or anything. Actually, it was like nothing I've ever felt before, but it was a sensation that you could feel inside your head, like a little twinge kind of thing. So then they put me back down and I woke up on my way to intensive care and that was pretty much all I can tell you about the brain surgery except that I heard a Dido song playing over and over again in my head and the doctors assured me they hadn't played any music in the surgery room, and I felt a comforting presence like a light, but also like a warmth or something like that. It was calming and soothing so I didn't freak out during the situation."

So Taylor was to be out of the hospital the next day, in a hotel room with Pam at the University Inn across the street, but still under care at Duke. The next day she called me again.

"We got the pathology back and Friedman is working out an aggressive game plan. They didn't get the whole tumor."

I remember asking her why not.

"To get it all would have damaged vital tissue. Mom mentioned something about doing my treatment up here. If anything, that would be detrimental to my mental health, Dad, to be out of my element and away from my support systems. Since it is mind over matter anyway, every little bit counts. I know I can beat this, Dad. I know I can."

Taylor was a social butterfly, but in a very serious way it was her peer group and her boyfriend that kept her going. To be among them was to be alive, to be with a future; that's what she meant. To be away from them would be to be away from life and she wasn't ready to be away from life.

I thought about the story of the train engine I had read to Taylor often when she was little. "I think I can, I think I can, I think I can." Taylor was the little brain tumor patient that could. But it was a pretty damn high hill to climb, I realized.

"It's going to be a bitch though," she said and then added. "Sorry for the language, Dad."

There was something else that went on during brain surgery, something that we discussed later, something Taylor couldn't explain: the comforting presence. She went into more detail about it.

"Dad, I felt there were two men in the room with me during the operation, and I had a feeling that I was going to make it."

"Who?"

"I'm not sure, but I think grandpa was there."

"Grandpa Joe?"

"I think so."

My former father-in-law, Joseph Coddington, had been dead a number of years.

I remember saying, "That's interesting,"

"There was someone else, I didn't know him."

"Who?"

"I don't know, he wasn't familiar to me," she said.

"You have no idea?"

"Not really, Dad."

"Nothing?"

"He might have had light hair."

I remember the cold shiver I felt when she told me this: could it have been *my* father? Taylor's paternal grandfather whom she had never met, Newton Black, died in 1974, nine years before Taylor was born. Were both of her grandfathers there in the room somehow to give her comfort? I believe strongly in God, but were her grandfathers her angels during that operation? Out of place and out of time, but I guess time is more for mortals, not for spirits. To this day, I can't explain it. Perhaps it was a hallucination, but if so, why would Taylor hallucinate about a man she never met?

I would fly up the next day, but I wouldn't meet Dr. Friedman. As fate had it, Taylor was released and we dashed to the airport to catch a flight back to Florida from Raleigh-Durham to avoid the hordes coming to Florida for the Super Bowl. But Taylor and I would return to Duke for the stem cell harvest a few weeks after that.

Still, to this day, I wonder, was my deceased father with my daughter during her second brain surgery? And if so, how was that possible?

Someday I will ask Taylor.

Taylor's Diary
July 5, 2001

Clouded thought fogs my mind.
I attempt to navigate the mist,
Unsure of my destination and the path that will lead me
there.
Is my endpoint not of this world?
What should I think of the journey?
I have turned on auto pilot and now it's stuck.
I struggle to regain control, not knowing where to begin.
Everything falls apart at once, I am speeding to the ground
in flames.
Frantically searching for a parachute I find none.

Chapter Thirty-Six: Diminishing Dreams

So, you are still trying to get my story published?

Yes, Taylor.

After all these years?

Uh huh.

You always were persistent, Pops, that's for sure.

I'm a mule, Taylor, and I want to get it right before I go.

Are you going somewhere?

You know.

Everyone's going where I've gone, Pops, but you don't know when that's going to be. No one does. How's that old song you sang to me once, "Oh Sweet Mystery of Life." Or something like that.

I sang that to you?

You sang a lot of songs to me when I was little. Remember Mom said she thought I'd marry a cowboy.

Yes, I remember that. I sang you a lot of country and western songs, that's for sure. You smiled a lot when I sang those.

I might have had gas, Pops.

No, I think it was the cowboy songs.

You like to think so, don't you? Well, I did fall in love with a boy who was going to be a NASCAR driver. Kind of a cowboy I think. NASCAR. Cowboys with cars instead of horses.

Yes, I would say so. Lot of horsepower there.

Bad pun, Pops.

Yeah, it was.

So what's the problem, Pops? You're down.

I'm not dreaming about you as much as I did.

I've been gone a long time, Pops. That's natural.

I feel guilty about it.

You shouldn't. Our memories fade like the ending of a movie when they roll the credits. They all fade to black

I still wonder if there was something else we might have done, something else we might have tried.

There wasn't. You did what you could. So did Mom. So did the Friedman boys at Duke. So did everyone. It's not your fault. I thought you were going to go with the alternating journals, Pops, your diary entry followed by my diary entry. I liked that concept. I thought that was really us.

It was, but the literary powers that be, said no one buys memoirs in the journal format anymore.

So something like The Diary of Anne Frank is passé?

It seems so.

I guess people don't have the patience for that form anymore. I suppose you have to do what you have to do.

Yes.

The "waves" are gone, aren't they, Pops? Those rushes of grief that would come over you when you drove to school in the morning and you would sob all the way to the parking lot?

Yes.

And you feel guilty about that too?

Yes.

Guilt is overrated, Pops. No one can keep up grief forever. Only Charlie Brown, I guess, with his "Good Grief," but he's a cartoon character. It was wise of you to seek counseling at Hospice with that counselor one-on-one. Too bad others in the family didn't do that.

You've finally let go. You know, that was the best advice you ever gave me, Pops.

What was that?

To let go and let God.

When did I say that?

At Martin Memorial a few days before I left, and we all knew I was going to leave, and you suggested I put myself in God's care. You surprised me.

Why?

I never thought of you as religious.

It wasn't religious, Taylor, it was spiritual.

We don't get so caught up in semantics here, Pops. Religious, spiritual. God, Allah, Jehovah, a rose by any other name.

Would smell as sweet?

Uh huh. Religious. Spiritual. Here they mean the same thing. I mean "I am who I am," right?

So are there trellis works there with little angels on the molding?

Huh?

You said you saw heaven when you were seven and there was a trellis with little cherubs atop the thing.

I did, didn't I?

Yes. So was that correct?

You'll have to find out for yourself, Pops. I don't do "trailers" to borrow a movie term.

I think I'll dream about you tonight, Taylor.

Yes, Pops, I think you will. "We are such stuff as dreams are made on; and our little life is rounded with a sleep."

Shakespeare?

The Tempest, Pops. But your life doesn't have to be one.

Taylor's Diary
July 14, 2001

CANCER!!! They said as it smacked me in the face,
TUMOR IN HER HEAD, THERE IS NOT TIME TO
WASTE.
CUT HER OPEN LET'S TAKE A LOOK
LET'S SEE HOW MUCH OF HER BRAIN IT TOOK.
POISON HER BODY, LET'S SEE WHAT THAT DOES.
ERASED ALL THE GIRL THAT SHE ONCE WAS.
MAKE HER SICK EVERY DAY, TIRED EVERY NIGHT,
IF SHE REALLY WANTS HER LIFE, WE GOTTA SEE
HER FIGHT.
Bring on the battle, bring on the foe. A gruesome war I shall
prevail I know.
Weak and weary, I'll battle to the death, try though it may it
won't take my breath.

Chapter Thirty-Seven: Hair

The week after the *60 Minutes* program aired in April 2002, a few teachers at my high school came up to me and said, in confidence, that they too had lost a child. It was as if I had just been initiated into some very secret society for those parents only seemed to talk about their loss with someone who could understand what it was like.

Reading Taylor's diary from June 2001, I remembered we still had high hopes as we set off for that last visit with "Nana," Taylor with her "hair" in hand.

On the way to my mother's from the airport in a rental car, Taylor took off her "hair," put a bandana over her baldness and turned on the radio and heard Ace of Bass's "The Sign" on an oldies station. It was Taylor's favorite song one year, years before, and it brought back memories to her of when she was little. "I'm amazed I liked that song so much, Dad," she said. "But I was just a kid."

"Just a kid." She had just graduated from high school and here she was talking about when she was "just a kid."

We drove on U.S. Route 30 through the metropolis of Wayne, passing the hair-dresser where Taylor went with her grandmother when Nana had her hair done on Saturday mornings. Nana loved to show off her granddaughters at the hairdresser, and then spoil them with a Dairy Queen ice-cream cone across the street. We passed the railroad station where the girls and I picked up the train for our Philadelphia excursions to the Art Museum, made famous, ironically, by the movie *Rocky* and the Franklin Museum, a wonderland of science geared toward children, where Taylor first walked through a larger than life replica of a heart. Those were what the poets call, the halcyon days.

We drove on past the Valley Forge Military Academy and wound ourselves around the tree-lined roads, and turned onto Knox Road and climbed the hill that lead to Valley View Lane.

When my parents bought the house a few years before my father died, a resident of Valley View Lane could actually see the valley below. But in the decades since my parents moved in, the growth of the trees had erected a verdant curtain and the valley was only visible in the winter season when the trees resembled wooden skeletons awaiting the leafy rebirth of spring.

"Dad, can you stop before we get there?" Taylor asked. "I have to put on my hair."

By "hair" she meant, of course, "wig," but oddly she seldom used the term "wig," except in her journal. Indeed, the "wig" was natural hair, a gift of an incredible neighbor, Patricia Jordan, who in many ways had been a surrogate mother to Taylor since she was a three-year-old. Pat was Katie's mother and Pat had asked me once to take Katie and Jamie for the weekend as their oldest daughter was in the hospital in Miami. Four little girls for a weekend was no big deal. I had slumber parties for Taylor and more kids than that. I don't know how many single fathers host slumber parties for eight or nine girls, but all the mothers treated me as if I was one of them, and I suppose I was a bit ahead of the curve back then. They nicknamed me "Mr. Mom."

Taylor, "hair" in place, was ready to meet her grandmother.

Nana knew nothing of Taylor's brain surgery. My mother was beginning the process of "the long goodbye" as President Reagan once commented about his own condition, and my brothers and I had hired a geriatric specialist who arranged for a woman to stay with my mother 24 hours a day.

Taylor had to make the decision as to whether or not to tell Nana of her condition. It was hard to see my mother in such a state. She had been such an active person. She was involved with the crisis telephone hot-line called "Contact" and she taught English to exchange professors' wives at the University of Pennsylvania. Much to my father's surprise when he arrived home from the office, my mother would have a Korean, Japanese or Indian couple sitting at the dinner table and I would learn something about the culture of their country as I ate my supper. But now it was obvious that this articulate woman was no longer "there."

I retreated to the downstairs family room, which became my nest when I visited my mother. My daughters would commandeer my bedroom which was next to my mother's. In 1987 when my marriage was going south and I had gone north to my mother's, I drank quite a bit of the booze she had on hand in my father's bar which was the prominent feature in the family room, my father being of the double shot of Canadian Club on the rocks type and a borderline alcoholic who hadn't lost his amateur status. After that little sojourn as a sot, I sought help from a renowned recovery program, but for the next ten years when a sober son visited his mother, alcohol was absent from the bar. My behavior in 1987 reminded her of the nights when she was a girl and had had to put her drunken father to bed. It was truly a surprise when, ten years later, she trusted me enough to return the liquor to my late father's bar. One visit, in my 7th year of sobriety, my mother asked me to take the garbage out to the cans in the garage, and I popped the lid on the wrong garbage can and, what-do-you-know, there were all the bottles from the bar. I never mentioned to her that I found the bottles by mistake and she went to her reward unaware of that fact, but I have told that story over to other recovering folks and it never fails to get a laugh. I was actually sitting in my father's old Lazy Boy remembering all of that when, after about thirty minutes with her grandmother, Taylor descended to the family room and announced, "I've decided not to tell Nana. It'll only confuse her."

It was a sad but practical decision for Taylor to make, I realized, and Taylor would write about it in her journal a day later, as included earlier in this volume.

I write to you from my Nana's attic, one of the most comforting places in the world for me. I always thought, If there is one thing that is constant in the world it is my Nana's home in Wayne, P.A. *I have come to the conclusion that there is nothing constant in this crazy world. I have not seen my Nana in 3 years, up until now. She has aged a lot in that time. She has a sweet woman that lives with her now and helps her out. She still knows what's going on but sometimes she is a bit forgetful. Enough so that we have not told her about my disease. It would confuse and frighten her. Hell, it confuses and frightens me! So, needless to say I have spent the majority of my stay peeking around corners to see if I need to put my wig back on before she saw me. But it is a pilgrimage that I needed to take in light of the past year I've had. I needed to find solace and retreat once more to my comfort zone. What I found here was change, which only reiterated the fact that I need to move forward and start anew. Having said that, our trip concludes on Sunday and I leave for Orlando on Monday. And so begins "Chapter 2: The Disney Years."*

I suppose the last trip to her grandmother's had taught Taylor that the only thing certain in life is change. It was part of the concept of "bittersweet" for that was the "bitter" part of the trip, the recognition of a verity. The sweetness was the amusement that Taylor and I shared in her "hair."

She and I took turns sitting next to my mother in her den as she sat like a zombie watching cable television. There would be lucid moments, of course, but for Taylor it was difficult because Nana confused her with her other grandchildren. When Taylor's hair became a bit hot, she would descend to the family room and I would take my post beside my mother in a version of the changing of the guard. That way, Taylor could take off her "hair" and have some peace without having to act for Nana's sake. One night Nana insisted that Taylor sleep in the second bed in her room, and poor Taylor's noggin was confined to the wig for the entire night. Even the woman who looked after my mother didn't catch on to Taylor's subterfuge with the hair.

The sum total of our visit was only three days, for in the words of Benjamin Franklin,

"Fish and visitors smell in three days" and Taylor and I packed our bags, said our goodbyes, and when we were out of sight of my mother's house at the end of Valley View Lane, Taylor exhaled and took off her 'hair'.

"I'm glad we came, Pops," she said.

"Nana is in bad shape, Taylor."

"I know. It's sad. But we were right not to tell her. Promise me you never will."

I remember answering "of course" but I wonder now what she was really trying to say to me. We would keep that promise to Taylor, and my mother would die about a year after Taylor did, not knowing her granddaughter would be there to meet her. But that's what Taylor wanted, and we honored her wishes.

Taylor's Diary
August 7, 2001

I haven't written in quite some time. I guess it's just a lack of action in my life. I have been doing the chemo pills & amazing enough it's true that these ones don't mess w/hair growth. I have a little bit of hair peeking through. These pills aren't event close to the IV chemo I was getting. Temodar is a walk in the park next to those. I have gotten sick a couple of times from them but it was nothing that I couldn't handle. Well, I start UCF in 13 days and I move into the new place on the 16th.

Well, what else is new? In the past month I have been doing a bit of traveling. I went up to see Jeff in N.C. for about 4 days. And then just recently I went to Atlanta. Both trips were wonderful. In the latest on the cancer front I started to see my doctor in Orlando; Dr. Nick (I can't pronounce his last name, Avergoloporus sp?). He is a very nice man & using my very refined radar I can tell that he is a good doctor.

The American Cancer Society asked me to speak @ a conference they're having the day after the scholarship luncheon. I'm nervous but sometimes it makes me feel better to express this rollercoaster ride w/a roomful of complete strangers. Lately I have been anxious. I'm not sure why, but it just sits there hanging over me. It's an accumulation of everything I think. My life has been drastically altered in this past year and it will never again be the same. I'm supposed to be carefree. I'm not supposed to worry about taking pills, eating right and getting enough rest. That's what you do when you grow up. Not now. I'm not supposed to have a bald head and tubes hanging out of my chest. I'm supposed to have long locks and a good tan. Why didn't this happen for me? Why do I have to be different? The woman from 60 Minutes called. She says that my story comes across too rosy, not enough pain & suffering and she'd like me to film the harder parts of it. For heaven's sake does the woman want to film me puking? Or maybe I should just go through another brain surgery so they can film that. FUCK THEM.

When that woman has been through what I've been through, then she can tell me what comes across is rosy. Until then, they can take their cameras & shove it where the sun doesn't shine.

There seems to be some stigma w/cancer. It seems that once you get it the world expects you to lie in bed and wait to die. And that will be just the thing that kills you. To heal, you have to truly believe you will and not let it take over your life. Make it as little a part of your life as you possibly can. I'm not saying ignore it. Just don't let it consume you. Fight the bastard until the bitter end. Because that's what it *is: a BASTARD. I really don't believe cancer is the right word for this disease. It doesn't mean enough. But, I suppose cancer is preferable because the word <u>can</u> is sitting right there & that alone gives you hope or at least it gives me hope.*

Taylor's Diary
August 8 2001

This is not a role I chose for myself,
Bald, sickly and pale.
All the things I was not I have become.
Forced to be the person you see now.
With the wounds of battle still apparent
And some not so.
I forge ahead, taking on this role to the best of my capability.
Thinking all the while: this does not suit me.
This is not what I was made for,
And then the daunting thought: perhaps it is.

Chapter Thirty-Eight: Commencement

Retired former teacher colleague Dick Sievenen and I were sitting together in the upper deck stands at the gym at Martin County High School, "Home of the Fighting Tigers," while down below our daughters—born three hours apart at Martin Memorial Hospital—were walking in to the packed room to the strains of Pomp and Circumstance.

"Commencement," the word actually means a beginning, but for the adolescents in caps and gowns marching to their rows of folding chairs for the graduation ceremony, this night meant only an end to high school and each and every one of them felt like Ferris Bueller on his day off.

Dick and I, as fathers, had a bond because of the coincidence of our daughters' births and so it seemed logical to sit next to him and away from Taylor's siblings and her mother. When the music stopped, Mikayla, Taylor's niece, called out "Tay Tay" to Taylor below, and Taylor smiled at her niece and put a finger to her lips in a "shhhh" sign. Meanwhile a cameraman lurked by Taylor, the ever-invasive CBS eye of the program *60 Minutes* which had sent a cameraman to capture Taylor's graduation on film.

"Courtney didn't go to her graduation," I said to Dick. "But Taylor wouldn't miss it for the world."

Courtney would go on to skip four graduations: high school, junior college, undergraduate and graduate. Taylor only got one chance at a graduation and it was a big deal to her.

"I'm so glad I can walk with my class, Dad," she said to me a few days before the ceremony.

"I didn't know it meant that much to you," I said.

"It's my friends, Dad, and our last time to be together."

It was more the party afterward than the ceremony, I realized, the alcohol-free party that the YMCA put on all-night after commencement. Merchants in town donated prizes which were raffled off for the students who attended, and the highlight was a new car provided by a local car dealer. The after graduation party had saved more than a few lives over the years as the students no longer felt the need to have keg parties after commencement.

I had asked Taylor about the all-night party.

"Do you think you can handle the party all-night, Taylor? Won't you be exhausted?"

"It can't be as exhausting as chemotherapy, Dad," she replied.

I could only smile.

After Taylor's name had been called early in the alphabetical roll call of graduates, a CBS cameraman came up to the upper deck of the gym where we were seated. I noticed the women in the family grabbing their compacts and checking their hair like so many Gloria Swansons at the end of *Sunset Boulevard* getting ready for their close-up from Mr. DeMille. I even realized that I had been running a comb through my own hair, not that it did any good. But the cameraman only smiled at us and pointed his camera down at the graduates, zooming in on Taylor, I assumed. Taylor was the star, we were only the extras.

Taylor's graduation was a hopeful sign for all of us. This was a normal progression. She had graduated from high school and now she was going off to college. In a few weeks she would be moving in with Gia and Karly and going to community college in Orlando. The doctors at Duke had said to "go on and live your life, Taylor," and at the end of May, 2001, it seemed like maybe, just maybe, she might beat the brain tumor. The new chemo was mild and seemed to be working, and that at least was hopeful as I watched her from the stands. She sat in a folding chair below me, she was all smiles and her "hair" was working perfectly and was securely on her head.

Commencement: it means a beginning, but, in retrospect, for, Taylor, it was the beginning of the end.

Taylor's Diary
August 10, 2001

As I run my fingers through my hair, the clumps begin to fall,
And as the hair hits the floor I am freed
Though I do not know it yet,
All that I knew of myself has been washed away,
My page is clean to write a new fate,
One of doctors and drugs
Surgeries and sickness.
One of strength.

Chapter Thirty-Nine: Grandchildren

In my dream Taylor and Jeff appear to be about thirty. They are sitting in their Florida room admiring the well-trimmed and decorated Christmas tree, one that Taylor has chosen as she was always the Christmas child. Two little children, a boy about two and a girl of four or five, both dressed in Disney pajamas, are rattling the presents beneath the tree, trying to discover just what is hidden beneath the fancy wrappings. Taylor is smiling at Jeff and then she sees me and says,

Do you like the name, Helen, Pops?

It is kind of old fashioned isn't it?

It was Nana's name.

She has your big brown eyes and your long brown hair.

She loves hats like I did.

Yes, you really loved to pose in your hats, didn't you?

So does she. The acorn didn't fall far from the tree.

It seldom does.

Yes, it seldom does.

So you named her after Nana?

Yes.

The boy looks like a terrible two, a terror in the making. He has a great little cowlick though, that's for sure. He looks like a Dennis the Menace in training. You named your son after Nana's maiden name?

Kane? Yes, although it is my middle name, remember. You gave me the same middle name as Courtney. Boy that was creative. Courtney Kane and Taylor Kane. I like Taylor though.

That was your mother's pick. I picked the middle names. She did all the work so she got to pick your first name. She named you after one of her favorite authors: Taylor Caldwell.

Never read him.

Taylor Caldwell was a her. I never read her either.

Gee, Pops, you were supposed to be my creative parent, the writer and all that, and yet you gave me the same middle name as Courtney. It's like I was a silly sequel or something. Kane II, the Sequel, coming to a basinet near you. You always said the only the only good sequel was The Godfather II.

I thought naming you with the same middle name as Courtney was different. Unusual. Unique even.

Sure, like George Foreman naming all his sons George. I'm surprised you didn't come out with a barbeque grill. The Kane-a-que.

It wasn't that bad. You named your boy after the family name "Kane." Why didn't you name him after Jeff?

We're not into the junior thing.

Beautiful children.

Aren't they, Pops?

I wish they could visit. I'd like to take them downtown to Hoffman's for some really good ice-cream.

That's sounds like what Nana always did with Courtney and me. The trips to Friendly's in Devon. Those were great times, Pops. Nana was an ice-cream addict. Every night for desert she fed us ice-cream.

Yes, those were the days. I miss those times.

I know, Pops. I know. We'll be back some other time, Pops. I promise.

Taylor's Diary
August 18, 2001

Well, I'm all moved in to my new apartment. All 3 of my roommates went home for the weekend but they'll be back tomorrow. They seem very nice. Tomorrow Henry calls me w/ the results of Mon.'s MRI. Let's keep our fingers crossed. 60 Minutes is sending a cameraman to film my conversation with Friedman. So, I have to wake up early.

In other news I registered for my classes. The times suck because I was the last group to register, but my classes are pretty decent. I have: Anthropology, Speech, Political Science and Musical Exploration (classical music).

That phone call from Friedman would tell Taylor that the MRI showed her tumor was another millimeter bigger, but it was nothing to be concerned about. But something was there and I certainly was concerned, as was Taylor, although she kept up appearances for the cameras. So it was to be two months for the new chem., then a return to Duke for observation in late October, but the best laid plans of mice and men and neuroncologists sometimes go astray.

Chapter Forty: The Irish Setter

Taylor's athletic career blossomed and ended on the volleyball court at Stuart Middle School with one magical season. In 8th grade she became a starter on the Stuart Middle School girls' volleyball squad and, being one of the more diminutive girls, she was selected as a "setter" or a player who "sets up" the ball for the taller and usually more athletic "spiker" whose job it was to smash the sphere over the net so that the opponents couldn't return it. Since Taylor was one quarter Irish, I nicknamed her "the Irish Setter" which she didn't seem to mind too much until it got a little old. Still, the position of setter was important as she was responsible for hitting the ball into the air at just the right height so the spiker could "spike" the ball at an angle which would make it difficult for the other team to return.

We had been through the gymnastic period a few years earlier after the ill-fated softball phase. Courtney was a good gymnast, but Taylor couldn't even manage an adequate forward roll. Somehow, when Taylor tried to do a forward roll she ended up sliding off the mat on her right shoulder, never quite completing the exercise. I didn't tell her, but I had had the same problem in gym class when I was a boy. I was a failure at the forward roll. I mean, let's face it, how many times in life is one going to need to do a forward roll? In the army I did quite a few "forward marches" but never forward rolls. It is really a useless exercise. Then again, how many times in life is one going to need to "set" the ball for a "spiker?"

But in 8th grade Taylor found her calling, and she was good at it and proud of herself for finally doing something successfully in the field of athletics. As a proud father I could see the future. She would go on to star at Martin County on Coach Marty Bielicki's storied volleyball team. Yes, the "Fighting Tigers" were among the elite volley ball teams in the state of Florida and had once been ranked among the Top 25 in *USA Today*. Then, after a successful career at Martin County, I envisioned a college scholarship for Taylor which would save dad some real money. After college, perhaps a coaching career. Who could foresee the future? My daughter had potential.

Unfortunately the Stuart Middle School team didn't. The Stuart Middle School girls lost more games than they won and yet Taylor was never depressed about the losses. She didn't seem to care if her team won or lost, even if there were no dandelions to pick. She was having fun just playing the game and being half-way good at it.

When the season ended we sat in the stands together and I discussed her future in volleyball.

"Are you going to try out for Mr. Bielicki's freshman team next year?" I asked her. "I think you could do it."

She looked at me as if I were daft.

"Are you kidding, Dad?"

"No. You have potential."

"I don't have a chance of playing for Mr. Bielicki."

Marty Bielicki and I had been colleagues for years and were good friends, but at that moment I wasn't above asking for a favor from him. "Sure you do," I replied. "I could make a phone call."

"No!"

I realized that such a phone call would be a mortifying embarrassment for her. "Okay, I won't. But don't you want to try?"

"Those girls are too serious about it, Dad. I like to play for fun. They're serious. It's not fun to them. It's like a job."

That was true. The serious volleyball players competed year round in "club volleyball," traveling all over the state and country to play against the best girls in the nation and hone their skills, all in hopes of a college scholarship. Dedicated parents tossed thousands of dollars into the "traveling teams" to make their daughters the best they could be. They were the athletic equivalent of beauty pageant girls whose parents managed their careers in hopes that Susie might land a modeling career because of a pageant. And with Title IX giving girls more athletic scholarships, there was a payoff to the girls who were good enough and dedicated enough to play volleyball.

Taylor wasn't one.

There were moments when I watched her play that I remembered my father. He had been a good athlete in college, winning a football scholarship to Shurtleff College in Illinois. He had always wanted his sons to be athletes like he was. My two older brothers had been disappointments so I was forced to play football, but for a baby fat boy who couldn't even manage a forward roll, how was I supposed to manage a forward pass. I made the kickoff team my senior year, but aside from kickoffs my posterior gathered pine splinters from the bench.

My father taught me one thing though. It didn't help for a father to press his child to participate in a sport in which he had only a modicum of talent. I resented my father for not letting me quit the team and I hated high school football, but after my discussion with Taylor, I was determined that we would never bring up the subject of high school volleyball again. I wasn't going to be my father, after all. She would hang up her knee pads after eighth grade and retire from the athletic world.

Taylor's Diary
August 26, 2001

Well, I have been here for a week and I must say I think my living situation will suit me well. My roommates are sweet and very easy to get along w/. This was definitely a good idea. I have to do work for some classes. I still have to write a speech for the American Cancer Society. I have a rough draft but it needs to be revised.

In other news, my chemo has been switched to a new one called VP16. I try to stay upbeat but I just wish we could find something that is visibly effective.

In all, I believe that I will really enjoy my classes this semester. I think that I'll be able to get a lot out of them. I think I'll get a lot out of this living situation also. I have discovered that through a bad situation more good will come out than you could ever imagine. Honestly, I believe. Let's hope that I can make some good also. I want to be proactive in my life. What's the point of pissing it away? That's what 99% of people do.

Chapter Forty-One: My Little Colonel

Early one Sunday morning, AMC was re-running a Shirley Temple film, *The Little Colonel* with Shirley playing a tantrum-prone Southern bellette who danced up and down a staircase with Bojangles Robinson. It reminded me of Taylor's dramatic period when she was the star of child-produced "movies" and I found the videotape of one of them, glad that I had recently decided on buying a machine with both VCR and DVD capabilities, for most of my videos of Taylor are on VCR cassettes.

I had, of course, remembered Taylor as a second Shirley Temple, and was a bit disappointed when I popped the tape to see that the productions were, how shall I say it, "childish?"

Taylor at 8 or 9 was hosting a make-believe formal dinner and greeting her friends as they came—overdressed—to Katie Jordan's bedroom door. Her long brown hair necessitated constant attention from her hand and she was forever pushing it back lest she wind up like some version of Veronica Lake.

Who's Veronica Lake, Pops?

Before your time, Taylor.

So were most things. Heck, my life was so short that there were a heck of a lot of things before my time and after my time. We were awful, weren't we?

I don't know.

Katie and Karly are so wooden in their acting. At least I seem a bit natural, don't you think?

Tracey taught you a few things, didn't she?

Tracey could act, Pops. Tracey could draw. Heck, Tracey is an artist.

You were a poet.

Maybe, I don't know. I mean I felt like I needed some type of creativity and you had taken the prose writing spot and Tracey had acting and Beth had painting. It's tough when you are the last kid.

I know. I was too.

Yes, we always had that in common didn't we?

You know, you reminded me of the Little Colonel when you were four or five. You threw some tantrums.

Yes, I was a brat. That video, boy I had long hair, didn't I?

A regular Rapunzel. You really liked to mug for the camera, Taylor.

Of course I did. I was half Mom, Pops, remember that. And the red head loved to show off, that's for sure. But it was you that made me pose for photos for your magazine articles.

You liked seeing your face in magazines and you were a tax write-off for the trips.

Gee, Pops, what did you used to say, I'm divorced and I have two tax write-offs?

You could have been a model.

Not when I went through my fat period unless I did the before for Jenny Craig. I was a real heifer.

Why did you like making plays so much?

Halloween, Pops. Remember how I liked Halloween? All kids like to dress up and be somebody different. That's why Halloween is so special to children, the candy is only secondary. For one night a child gets to be a goblin or a ghost or a movie star and not just a little kid that no one really listens to. Halloween is the ultimate in play and next to Christmas, Halloween was my favorite day of the year.

I remember that.

I never really got into Shirley Temple, Pops. No child could be that precocious, could she?

I looked at a photo of Taylor on the wall across the living room. She was perhaps ten, dressed in jeans and a jean jacket with a matching jean beret, looking like some Calvin Klein ad, giving a thumbs-up sign.

Yes, I thought, all children are precocious in their own special way. Then again, Taylor loved to play with her Barbies, often joining the Jordan girls in the make believe world of domestic bliss with Ken and Barbie, where Ken was the perfect husband and Barbie had the perfect hour-glass figure that probably contributed to an increase in anorexia and bulimia among the teenage girls who had been Barbie's buddies in pre-pubescence. Courtney never played with Barbies and I wonder if that had something to do with her choice of keeping her maiden name when she married.

That's really a stretch, Pops. Are you thinking that you might be the reason for Courtney's feminism?

I don't know.

Well, you weren't, Pops. You weren't responsible for my playing with Barbies either. Neither was Mom. Feminism means choices, Pops, and I would have been happy with a husband and children. A career for me would have been secondary. Courtney and I were different.

I realize that now.

But you treated us the same.

205

I guess I did.

Because your father said he treated you all the same.

Yes.

But he really didn't. He didn't force your brothers to play football did he?

No. He didn't.

Pops, you've got to let that football nonsense go. It was forever ago. And don't be so hard on yourself, Pops, or you will need a meeting.

Thanks, Taylor.

Let's go for a drive in the Tercel, Pops.

Good idea.

Taylor's Diary
August 27, 2001

A cleansing of the soul began in the absence of my hair
As though it had been a curtain shielding this beauty all
along,
Knowing all the while that I would never look,
Now stumbling upon it, and falling hard,
Smacked in the face by bittersweet wonder.
How did I never realize the paradise awaiting,
It's funny the way you realize,
By being hit by a hurling brick.

Chapter Forty-Two: Lance Armstrong

In the last year of her life, Taylor heard a great deal about cyclist Lance Armstrong and surely his story was truly inspirational, especially for cancer patients. Lance overcame testicular cancer, resumed his career as a cyclist, and went on to become Tiger Woods on a bicycle, winning a number of the coveted Tour de France trophies. From chemo to primo, one might say, but recently he returned to the Tour de France, coming out of retirement and finishing third. Not bad, I thought, for a has-been, and reading the sports section I thought of Taylor, not as a cancer patient this time, but rather as a beginner on her bike, the day we took the training wheels off.

I was teaching at Martin County High School and living across the street from the school in a duplex in a divorced dad development known as Hideaway Place, a catchy name for a place that wasn't such a hideaway, but rather a series of rentals for fathers who had visitation rights with their children. On weekends the street would be populated by an influx of kids, but by Monday they would be gone, along with a child support check, back to the bosom and the bank account of their mother.

For me, it was convenient, and one Saturday morning Courtney, Taylor and I with two bikes, walked across the main road to Martin County High School to the inside courtyard where I proposed to give little five-year-old Taylor her first lesson in driving under the influence of balance.

There was something reassuring for a little child in the training wheels on her bike. They seemed to aright the teetering of a tot in motion as she pedaled furiously down the driveway. This was a time before the obsession with children wearing helmets to ride their bikes. If a kid fell on his noggin, well, he fell on his noggin. In retrospect, it is amazing that anyone of my generation even survived childhood, having had lead pencils, no adult supervision at baseball games, no bike helmets, no seat belts, and a penchant for playing in the dirt. Every boy I knew in childhood was a clone of Pig Pen from *Peanuts*. But all of us, at one time or another, had had to cross the childhood threshold from training wheels to two wheeler, and I, for one, had a problem with the concept of brakes. As a child it made no sense to me that a cyclist had to suddenly pedal in the opposite direction if he wanted to stop. This, of course, was before the advent of ten speed bikes. I had a three speed Schwinn when I was a kid, and I thought I was the Cat's Meow, as most of the guys had the conventional one speed bike, and so did Taylor on that fateful day in the courtyard at MCHS.

In something of a small ceremony with Courtney watching, I applied pliers to the training wheels and removed them from Taylor's Strawberry Shortcake bicycle.

"There," I said when completed. "A two wheeler."

Taylor smiled, but I sensed apprehension behind the smile. I knew she was nervous, because she didn't say anything; Taylor was a chatterbox.

Still, courageously she took a seat on the bike, her little legs holding the bike securely in place.

"I'm going to push you to get you started, Taylor."

She nodded nervously.

Of course I was nervous, Pops, you forgot to tell me about the importance of the brakes.

You knew about brakes, Taylor.

Yes, but I was trying to maintain my balance and remembering brakes too was just too much for me to handle.

And you crashed into the glass door entrance to the courtyard.

It wasn't glass on the door; it had glass panels on either side, kind of skinny actually.

And you managed to whack right into one of them and break it. I yelled to you to hit your brakes.

Pops, I was five years old. I was a klutz. What can I say? I was no Lance Armstrong. Remember what Tristan said about Lance Armstrong when we were getting our stem cells harvested at Duke and that nurse tried to use Lance Armstrong and his autobiography as an inspiration for us?

Yes, I do. He said. "Big deal. We go through a Tour'd France every day." I liked that kid.

He had medulloblastoma, the brain tumor found in the base of your head by the brain stem. It had also spread to his spine. He had had it for thirteen months and had undergone chemo and radiation and two rounds of pheresis and was then doing more chemo. He was extremely good natured and courageous, and I admired him.

They once thought you might have had medulloblastoma.

Yes. Heck, they thought I had Glioblastoma too, the nasty stuff, but I think Tristan had an interesting take on the subject of Lance Armstrong. He said he thought Lance Armstrong got the best care possible because he was a celebrity. "What about average people?" I remember him asking asked the nurse. He had gone through a lot. He hadn't written a best seller, but he was a gutsy guy. I liked his goatee but the Cleveland Indians cap was kind of lame.

I think Lance Armstrong would have liked Tristan.

Probably, Pops. Didn't you get into a bit of trouble because of my bike accident, Pops? With Wanda Yarboro?

Wanda Yarboro was my principal then, and I was in her office Monday morning, telling her our story and offering to pay for a new glass panel. God bless her, may she rest in peace. She just laughed and said they would take the repairs out of the soda money receipts. They made money on the pop in the teacher's lounge.

You know, Pops, after that little accident I never had a problem with brakes or balance again, except in gymnastics I guess.

And the two broken arms.

Oh, I forgot about those.

We removed the cast from the first broken arm and within a month you had broken your other arm. Fell off a bleacher?

Brain tumor, Pops. Probably the brain tumor. Even then, that brain tumor was already messing up my life.

Taylor's Diary
September 11, 2001

Today is a day that will not be forgotten. This morning 4 commercial jets were hijacked. 2 flew into the World Trade Center Towers, collapsing them and causing mass chaos. And then, while I was watching the news the Pentagon was attacked. A 4th hijacked plane crashed near Pittsburgh. The tragedy of this day cannot be measured. It is certainly unprecedented. My heart goes out to the poor victims & their families. I pray for them and for our country.

Crash! One by one a nation hits the ground, blocking out the sun, no survivors can be found.

Screaming in the streets, panic in the parks, a gruesome day to mark.

And when the dust has cleared the tears begin to shed, the magnitude is realized through the dead.

Chapter Forty-Three: The Hardwood

At Duke University there is one intercollegiate sport that matters, the one played with a round ball on a hardwood floor: basketball. The men predominate in the game, but the women fill the gym with fans for their games as well, and Taylor had befriended Duke's star player, Georgia Schweitzer, who was a pre-med protégé of the doctors Friedman. Georgia, who was the epitome of a student athlete, met Taylor when she accompanied Henry Friedman on rounds at the hospital. Taylor, unnamed, became part of a diary which Georgia was compiling for a sports channel as I recall. The evening after Taylor's surgery for the correct pheresis line, Georgia left two passes for Taylor and me for the game with Florida State University.

In the recovery room after surgery to put in the proper line for the pheresis, the recovery room nurse suggested Taylor forgo the basketball game that evening to get some rest.

That wasn't going to happen, Pops. There was no way I wasn't going to go to that game. The thought of the game that night had made surgery bearable, that and beagles.

That's right; you talked to the physicians about dogs, especially beagles. That was an odd thing to talk about, Taylor.

I liked to talk to take my mind off what the surgeons were doing to my body, Pops. It was how I coped. That and having something to look forward to like the basketball game that night. I wanted to see Georgia play.

You gave the nurse the that-isn't-going-to-happen smile and didn't say a word when she told you shouldn't go the game.

You backed me up. You said we'd be going with my doctor, and the nurse got kind of huffy with you. You were a terrible parent, Pops.

Maybe, but I hadn't even met Dr. Friedman at that point as he wasn't directly involved with the pheresis. I certainly wanted to meet the head man in your case.

You know, Pops, you came into the recovery room and talked about the Protestant Reformation. That was kind of weird.

You might recall that we still had to get you through two courses for a high school diploma and I was serving as your homebound history teacher.

I remember. But it was still kind of silly. You gave me a B for the class too. Beth gave me an A for the sculpture class and I did more work for you.

I thought I shouldn't cut you too big a break, and the grade didn't matter anyway, you were in UCF. You would have given yourself a C.

No, Pops, I would have given myself a D, probably a D minus.

But you're right, Taylor. It was an improper time to discuss the Reformation.

Is there ever a proper time to discuss the Reformation, Pops?

You're going to make me laugh.

I hope so. You could use a laugh. Remember I won the bet about Henry's car?

Yes, we were standing outside of the University Inn and you said you figured he drove a Volvo, that Dr. Friedman was a Volvo kind of guy.

And what kind of car did he show up in?

A Volvo.

You didn't hit it off with Henry, did you Pops?

No. I didn't like him.

Because he didn't pay any attention to you?

I guess. I asked him a bunch of questions, but he never once asked me about my life. And I sat next to him in the stands.

Henry hurt your feelings. Poor Pops. Boo hoo. I liked him.

Yes, you liked him and he certainly liked you. I liked Alan Friedman though. He was friendly. He was so delighted that you weren't limping when you walked. You were limping before you went into his surgery. Henry's son was nice as well. He was taking an A.P. course.

You always got along well with kids, Pops. Maybe you were jealous of how well Henry got along with me.

You two had great rapport. You had great rapport with Georgia too. I remember calling you at UCF to turn on a TV because Georgia was playing on ESPN in the WNBA and she made a three point shot.

She was really nice to me, Pops, but she was depressed that night when Duke lost the game by two points.

Until she saw you come out of the crowd. When she saw you, her face brightened into a smile and I guess the game seemed secondary to her. You had that way about you, Taylor, you really did. You had a smile that would launch a thousand ships.

I'm sorry you didn't like Henry Friedman, Pops. I know you think he promised more than he delivered, but he really did his best. It broke him up when I passed. He takes his patients' deaths pretty hard sometimes.

I thought he was a 60 Minutes *showboat at times. That trip we made in October, the last one I made with you, the one that Tracey made as well, coming down from Richmond, and there we were before the cameras, you, Tracey and I. And the Friedmans were looking at your scans and telling us things weren't going quite as well as we had hoped and using the friggin' basketball analogy that it was the third quarter and you were down twelve points, that there was good news and bad news and the bad news was that there was no response to therapy and the good news was that you were going downhill slowly, that the bad news was there were no guarantees, but the good news was that there was more time to try options. And the shunt to the brain to pour the chemo directly on the tumor so they could shrink the tumor for stem cell. And Henry, like some Wizard of Oz, hinting that there was something that might be available in six months, and realizing there was only a man behind the curtain after all. But I remember your mom saying Henry called her and was truly upset when he learned the news in late November.*

You're not sorry that interview with you and I and Tracey at Duke didn't air on 60 Minutes?

No, I'm glad I was never on camera. I think they cut us out because they were able to film the results of that last operation in which they came into the hospital room to say the procedure hadn't worked, that those dead cells weren't a result of residue from radiation treatments.

You remember all of it, don't you, Pops?

Even these years later, in an instant I can be at Duke with you, in a conference with Henry Friedman or on the floor of 5200. It seems to be etched in the very core of my soul. I was watching the reports of the death of Teddy Kennedy and there it was once again, the entrance to the Duke University Hospital.

My home away from home, Pops. Didn't you find it interesting that Ed Bradley had cancer? That even during the program when he interviewed me he was suffering from cancer. I'm glad he won his Emmy. You root against Duke now, don't you?

Every game, Taylor. Every game.

Taylor's Diary
September 17, 2001

I haven't been writing anything lately because I haven't been doing much. Our country is preparing for war against an unknown enemy. It's a sad, sad time in history occurring right now. Everywhere you go you see American flags & signs saying "God Bless America." It gives me chills.

In other news I finished my 1st round of VP-16 chemo. I jinxed myself: on the last day of taking it I had said that it hadn't made me sick once (I didn't knock on wood). And wouldn't U know on the way to my Grandma's this weekend, I had to pull over and get sick. But, luckily I made it to Grandma's cause if there was anywhere I'd rather be since that is the best place.

Chapter Forty-Four: Swan Song

I was trying to remember the color of your bandana that you wore for that speech at the Swan Hotel ballroom, Taylor, two days before the attack on 9/11. The American Cancer Society convention?

The bandana was sky blue, Pops. So was the dress; it was a matching outfit. Mom helped pick it out.

Your mom was a shopper; she should have turned pro I thought. It was kind of ironic in a way, I suppose, because you had had a spinal MRI a few days before that and it was clear. But you were favoring your leg. Aunt Barbara noticed that. That was always an indication that the tumor was back. Watch the DVD with me. There's the cheesy music and the cheesy screen in the background with the wand and the logo, The Magic Touch.

C'mon, Dad, it was Disney. Mickey's a mouse. You have to expect "cheesy" stuff.

Shhh. The camera shows you limping a bit as you went on stage.

I was. Shhh.

"Today, I'd like to tell you about a story of hope. Once upon a time..."

I forgot you started with the fairy tale opening.

Shhh.

"...there was a young girl who was just like any other. She had long hair that flowed down her back and a healthy body. Her only worries consisted of Algebra homework and planning the upcoming weekend. And she was content. Until one night, when everything she knew and thought was changed forever.

'Mom, you're overreacting. My leg will be fine,' she pleaded.

'I don't like the look of it,' her mother replied. 'Let's take you to the hospital.'

'But, Mom, it's Friday night!'

'Well then, we better hurry if you want to go out with your friends.'

"And so the young girl went to the hospital, convinced her mother's paranoia had no merit.

"After a while a man came into the waiting room, wearing a white coat. 'All your tests are normal, we're just going to give you a CT scan and then you can all get out of here.'

"As the young girl headed to the room with the strange machine, she was wondering if she still had time to meet her friends, and thinking just how crazy her mother could be at times.

"After what seemed like hours of waiting, the doctor came in. 'Maybe you should sit down,' he said to them.

'What is it?' her mother shakily questioned.

"The 'cat' scan revealed a large mass on her brain. 'She is going to need emergency surgery.' The girl looked over at her mother, who looked as though she had just been hit by a speeding truck. 'This can't be true,' the girl thought. This happens to other people, people I don't know—not me!'"

Isn't that always the way we feel?

Shhh.

"As the girl tried to process this life-altering news a nurse came from behind with a wheelchair. 'Sit down, honey,' she said rather sorrowfully. 'I'm going to take you to a room and *we're going to start you on steroids to prevent any swelling.'"*

I never would have made it into the Hall of Fame, Pops.

Shhhh.

"Unable to think, the girl looked down at the medical chart in disbelief: Diagnosis:

Brain Tumor.

"For the next few hours the girl sat in the hospital bed, stunned, not really thinking anything, just wondering if this was real. After a while her mother returned with a few of her things and one of her brothers. 'Are you alright?' he said as he quickly came to her side.

'I guess so,' she numbly replied.

'Do you want me to call your dad?' her brother asked in a rather scared tone.

'Are you kidding me?' she replied. 'At this hour? That's the last thing I need to do. If he was awakened to this news, he'd surely have a heart attack. And I definitely do not need a dead father. No, I'll tell him in the morning.'"

I had forgotten your mother didn't even call me, Taylor. But it was good that you didn't tell me that night. I might have kicked the bucket, and I paid your medical insurance.

Shhhh.

"After the girl's brother left, she and her mother set up camp, finding relief only when their heads hit the pillows. As the girl awoke in the unfamiliar hospital room, one thought consumed her: How would she tell her father? How do you tell a parent that their worst fear had become a reality?"

You did that well.

221

"'Hey, what are you doing up so early?' her father cheerfully greeted her as she walked through the door.

'Sit down for a second, Dad,' she continued."

You thought it was a car accident, didn't you?

I didn't know what was coming. I never did with you. You were the surprising child. Shh, I want to hear your speech.

"'Is something wrong?' he asked, not wanting her to answer.

"As she explained to him all that she knew about her current situation, she could see the light in his eyes disappear. And when she was finished they both sat there, not knowing what to think. After a while her father responded, 'You can beat this,' he said confidently.

'I hope so,' she silently thought.

"In the weeks that followed the girl underwent emergency surgery and traveled to Duke University to ultimately be diagnosed with a cerebral neuroblastoma, a malignant brain tumor.

"It looked bad, real bad. The young girl was worried and resentful. 'Why me?' she thought. As she began chemotherapy, the fact that she would lose her hair soon came to fruition."

Nice word, "fruition."

Shhh.

"Her long brown locks quickly gave way to a shiny bald head. It was then that it happened: something inside the girl transformed and she realized how thoroughly unimportant hair was. She gained a new perspective on life and a freedom others could only dream about.

"The chemo began to take its toll, weakening her body but never her spirit. There were still times when she'd cry. But what seventeen-year-old girl wouldn't cry when faced with her own mortality? And when she was finished crying, she somehow knew that she was going to beat this disease.

"So she forged on through more chemotherapy, surgeries and radiation. She attended her high school prom. She graduated with her class. And with the help of the American Cancer Society she went off to college. Now a year later the young girl continues to fight, knowing that she will ultimately win. That girl's name is Taylor Black and that girl is me."

"I am that girl" would have been correct.

Always the teacher, Pops. Always the teacher.

No, Taylor, you were the teacher. I was the student...I was the student. And the class was Life.

* * *

On October 7, 2001 Taylor called from Orlando. She was in the Florida Hospital. What we had feared had transpired. She wanted nothing more than to spend her life helping others. I didn't want to lose her, but at that moment I had a foreboding. I asked God why, but He didn't answer.

I tried to tell myself, I must remember how fortunate I am. Thousands of innocent people were killed on September 11, but that only seemed surreal. Taylor was reality.

Taylor's Diary
October 15, 2001

Too much energy pulled from my veins,
For each new day's battle a drop more depletes
A fume for which I strain
As my heart just barely beeps.

Chapter Forty-Five: College Days

A week before fall 2001 classes started at the University of Central Florida, Taylor moved out of Gia and Karly's apartment and into a housing complex, sharing a large apartment with three other young women. Each woman had her own room, bathroom and shower, but there was a common living area and kitchen. After meeting her roommates, Taylor came out to the parking lot where I was unloading a car and gave me an enthusiastic hug: "They are perfect, Pops," she said.

It was the multi-cultural she was after. There was another white girl, but a Latina and an African-American gal as well. "I hit the jackpot," she said. "This is why I came to UCF, for the diversity."

Taylor and the black student named Celia worked out a deal. Taylor helped Celia with English in return for Celia tutoring Taylor in mathematics, and they became fast friends. And none of the other girls thought anything about Taylor's pot smoking for nausea. The other Anglo girl even passed along the information to her grandmother who was having nausea with her chemotherapy.

She got her grandmother some weed and the old lady smoked it, Pops. Kind of cool I thought.

Remember those last classes at UCF? We came back from Duke in mid-October and you were staying with your grandmother Virginia in Melbourne.

She made the most beautiful dolls. She was truly an artist, Pops. She even gave me one.

You couldn't drive at the time; it wasn't safe as we were afraid of a possible seizure. So I drove up from Stuart and picked you up and then drove you to Orlando for your classes.

Political science class. I was heavy on the steroids and eating like a horse.

I remember hanging out in the library while you were in class, trying to find old articles I wrote for the Miami Herald when I still thought I was going to be the next Ernest Hemingway. You had never read those family friendly stories I cranked out, funny little tales of life with your mother when she played Lucy to my Ricky, the days when our marriage actually worked, when we finished each other's sentences. But UCF didn't have the Herald on microfilm and the pieces were too old to have been put on the internet archives.

You found a couple of magazine articles, Pops. The Sunta Claus one. I really liked that one. How you and Mom hired a Rent-a-Santa when we were little. Face it, Pops; the red head gave you a lot of material for articles. There can be a gold mine in dysfunction.

She could put the "zip" in Zippidy do-dah, alright. I remember the ride back to Melbourne that night, Taylor, and I remember we taped our conversation.

For our diaries, Pops. We were going to publish our diaries when I beat cancer. It was going to be a best seller and Sally Field would play mom in the movie version and Julia Roberts would play the twins because they look just like her.

I remember you working on the casting for the movie. I wanted to be played by Robert Redford.

That was amusing, Pops. Robert Redford as you. If he gained forty pounds.

Cruel, that's cruel. But that night on the ride back from UCF you said something interesting.

You mean when I spoke of cancer patients and how we thought? I can quote myself:

"This is something big. I don't know. Something that's indescribable. It's already been life altering. It's like a different level of consciousness we're on than everyone else. A more pure life. Real. It's not just stuff—I can't exactly put my finger on it."

The concept of facing death was what it was, Taylor. The idea was with mortality staring you in the face you didn't have time to blink.

It was a spiritual awakening, Pops, that's what it is and you have that in your program as well. Remember in the hospital when I said, "there's a reason for all of this, Pops. I just hope it's grand?"

Yes, you knew you were dying at that point in time. You were turning it over to God. You know, your mother doesn't believe you ever said that.

That's too bad. I did.

It was grand, Taylor. It was grand.

I like to think so. Every life is grand in its own way.

We played the Beatles tape that night in the car and it reminded you of all the trips on the interstate to Nana's.

The Beatles One album. Courtney and I bought you that for Father's Day, Pops. All their number one hits. And I talked about how much I had eaten that day because of the steroids. A bagel with crème cheese and two blueberry muffins, a few bananas and a cup of pudding for breakfast. Then potato chips for snack. Then lunch of clam chowder, shrimp salad, lots of bread and presidential chocolate cake. Then two six inch turkey subs, a super-size fry and a milk shake. *I was due to have another operation a few weeks later at Duke to put in the Rickham Reservoir in my head and I was going to be under general anesthesia, therefore it would be impossible for me to eat for a week, so I packed on extra pounds. That was the reason I looked like a heifer.*

You always referred to yourself as a heifer.

I felt like one. Big as a cow because of the steroids. Of course I don't have a weight problem now. Daydreams don't need to go to Jenny Craig.

No they don't, Taylor. No, they don't.

Taylor's Diary
October 16, 2001

Sleep and peace please come to me, I beg of you just this.
Erase my memory with your unconscious kiss.
Take me in your arms, let thoughts escape my head,
Keep away all harm and any tears I've shed.
Let me now just rest for a moment more,
Release me from the stress that stands beside my door.
Rock me soft and gently through the darkest hours of night
Awaken me to morning's healing light.

Chapter Forty-Six: One Day in Anatomy Class

Going through some things in Taylor's old bedroom, I came across a thank-you card addressed to Taylor and signed by the students in the Anatomy and Physiology class at South Fork High School. Some of the students, the girls of course, wrote little notes of appreciation. The boys, characteristically, merely signed their names.

It was August of 2001 and South Fork had begun its semester a few weeks ahead of the college opening and Taylor had some time on her hands. I can't remember whose idea it was but one morning Taylor came to school with a number of brain scans to show the students what a brain tumor looked like on a CT scan.

She dropped by my portable classroom to say hello, but I couldn't leave to hear her speak as I had a class at the same hour as Anatomy and Physiology. The science teacher, Ms. Schumacher, was a veteran, no-nonsense teacher of the old school with thirty years of experience in the classroom and yet that day she was moved by Taylor.

I was good, Pops. The kids were really interested.

Many of them showed up in my later classes that day and told me how amazing you were.

I was, Pops. I was. I was really "on" that day. It was one of my good days.

Stop smiling. You are not supposed to have an ego in the afterlife. Don't laugh at your father, that's not polite. As I was saying the kids were amazed by your positive attitude more than the brain scans.

They found them interesting though, Pops. I taught them how to read a scan and what the doctors looked for. I told them of my brain operation at Duke and how I was awake about half of the time. I think by that time the Discovery Channel had already done a show on brain tumors where the patient was awake. The kids were really interested, more than I was when I was in high school.

Oh, like you hadn't graduated from high school only three months before that?

I don't know, Pops, it was odd. I felt so much older than the kids. They were juniors in high school, only two years younger, but I felt much older than they were. I felt older than kids my own age, come to think of it.

The last year was a maturation I couldn't believe.

That was the good part.

The students in that class were upset three months later when you died.

Not as much as I was, Pops.

Don't smile like that. That wasn't funny.

Why not smile, Pops; I'm in a better place. There's no homework here. I don't have to clean my room or worry about what I'm going to wear for a date. Or be concerned that I have overdrawn my checking account.

Some of the students from that class showed up at the funeral home for the service we had there, the night before your funeral.

I'm glad you had a black priest, Pops.

Your mom's the Catholic, not me. It was her pick.

Nice crowd though. Lots of students. The death of a child really packs them in, doesn't it?

Your grandfather was president of an international labor union but you had more people show up for your funeral than showed up for his.

That's what he told me. He wasn't jealous though. He was happy you turned out to be a teacher, Pops. That's what he wanted to be until the Great Depression cost him his football scholarship and forced him to drop out of college.

There it is, football again. I've got to let it go. I believe the Anatomy teacher taped the 60 Minutes program and showed it to the students.

That would complete the circle, Pops. For some of those kids, I might have been the first person they met who actually died. I would think that was a pretty powerful lesson, wouldn't you?

Yes, yes I would, Taylor.

Then it was worth it.

Taylor's Diary
October 17, 2001

I want to cry a thousand tears, but my eyes won't muster
one,
I want to drown my fears and wash away the sun.
I want it all to cease, the breathing, hurt and pain.
I need to have release from the pounding of the rain.
I want to scream at decibels my voice could never go,
I must have someone come and take away this low.

231

Chapter Forty-Seven: Amish Country

Like many single men, I know I'm not much of a housekeeper. Dust bunnies have hutches in my house and piles of rejected novels clutter the coffee and end tables, constantly reminding me of my literary failings. But on occasion, when I'm expecting company of the opposite gender, I put my hand to housecleaning, especially dusting off the pictures around the house.

One day, expecting company, I was dusting the pictures and removed one of my favorites from its spot on my bedroom wall and wiped its glass covering: Courtney and Taylor were posing in a cornfield, sticking their heads between the corn stalks, smiling at the camera. It reminded me of Nana and Amish Country.

Nana loved Amish Country, Pops. But we loved it that you split your pants.

That's right. Boy that was embarrassing. It was a good thing I was wearing underwear and I wasn't going commando.

That's Joey from Friends, Pops. You stole that.

Yes I did. We had just ridden the old railroad at East Stroudsburg and when I detrained I split my pants. I had to stop and get another pair.

It's amazing that the highlight of that trip was split pants. Nana got sort of nostalgic in the one room Amish school house.

She taught in one in Illinois in the 1930s. For two years I think it was. Until she married my father.

And lost her job.

Yes, she liked to tell that story. That Illinois county that hired her dismissed women teachers when they married. Only spinsters were allowed to teach.

I guess I was a spinster, wasn't I?

You were eighteen. Spinsters didn't become spinsters until their twenties in the old days.

There are so many negative names for women, Pops. Spinster is one. Old maid is another. Single men are merely bachelors. It's not fair.

No it isn't.

Nana really liked to teach, Pops. She talked about it so often and she only taught for two years. That was really a shame that she couldn't teach because she got married. Her whole generation was subservient to their husbands.

Yes, that's the way it was, Taylor. Nana was a great grandmother wasn't she?

I loved going to see her, Pops. She spoiled me rotten. We did so many day trips with you and her. We did the Amish country three times and you only split your pants once.

I'm glad you remembered more than that.

I always liked the cornfield photo, Pops.

I nearly gave that to you when you went off to college, Taylor, but I thought it would be corny to do so.

Ha ha, Pops.

No one laughs at my puns any more, Taylor.

Courtney never cared for them. Only I did. So did Karly Walker. She loved your puns, Pops.

She's teaching in St. Petersburg.

No, she's in California now, we chat.

Tracey Jordan in Colorado saw you in her bedroom one night.

I think I frightened her. First time. You know Nana's house reminded me of something Maya Angelou once wrote.

You loved Maya Angelou.

Uh huh, she wrote, "The ache for home lives in all of us, the safe place where we can go as we are and not be questioned." That was Nana's for me.

I know, Taylor. Give her my love.

I will, Pops. I will.

Taylor's Diary
October 19, 2001

I cannot breathe. The more I try the more I gasp. HELP!
DOES ANYONE SEE ME HERE?
DOES ANYONE SEE ME CHOKING?
FREE ME! GIVE ME AIR. HELP ME. JUST A BREATH!
JUST ONE LIFE SUSTAINING FORCE! GASP

BLACKNESS!

Chapter Forty-Eight: Death Be Not Proud

Back in the late 1940s, journalist John Gunther wrote a book about his son Johnny's fight with brain cancer. The book, entitled *Death Be Not Proud,* has never been out of print. It is a timeless classic, and although John Gunther wrote several best sellers such as *Inside the U.S.A* and *Inside Europe,* his biography of his son is the one which has stood the test of time. I reread it recently and it took me back to Taylor's last days and to her last journal entries.

And as it turned out, Courtney was in Orlando as she had snuck away from the University of Florida to fly to Las Vegas to catch a Stevie Nicks concert. *Your daughters were always surprising you, Pops. Read from my journal, Pops, the October 28, 2001 entry. It was after your last trip with me to Duke, from my point of view:*

Taylor's Diary
October 28, 2001

Well I haven't kept up with writing because my life was going pretty smoothly up until three weeks ago. Then I started to get headaches and get nauseous one day, and I called Dr. Nick and he made me stay in the hospital overnight and they gave me an MRI and discovered the cancer leaking down into the CSF (cerebral spinal fluid). I had to get a spinal tap. That was NOT FUN! And now I am up at Duke, doing a new treatment. I just got something called a Rickham Reservoir. This will act kind of as a port. They will administer a new "test" chemo through that and it will go everywhere the cancer cells are going. Doctors Friedman (Henry and Alan) gave me an analogy that we are in the third quarter and are down by 12. They are all about basketball here and 12 points aren't that much. But it's definitely a B-I-T-C-H. I keep wondering if I will eventually die from this. I'm gonna try as hard as I can but what if I don't have it in me? I'm trying to muster up every piece of strength and energy I have right now. I start treatment on Tuesday. It is apparently a four hour procedure so I'd better bring a book. I am going to keep you updated along with my 5 million relatives who are driving me a very short trip to crazy. Until then.

Yes, their slogan was "At Duke there is hope." For a while after everything that occurred, I thought it was, "At Duke there is hype." As if we were promised a cure that never came, that sort of thing. I'm just reading from your own diary from November 12, 2001.

That was my last diary entry, Pops. There wasn't really much to write after that, was there?

No, I guess not.

Taylor's Last Diary Entry
November 12, 2001

Well, we have a minor setback. This new chemo is not as effective as we would have hoped, so we have to switch to a different one. Let's keep our fingers crossed TIGHT!

I think it upset the family more than me! Of course I was extremely bummed out, but what are you gonna do? Really what can you do? The most precious gift is life and working for it will only make the reward that much sweeter in the end. I truly am a blessed individual in so many fantastic ways. I need to always remember my infinite blessings in the time that the "oh, poor me syndrome" overwhelms me. It's a long hard road but the pot at the end of the rainbow is more than all that the leprechauns in all the world could ever have hoped 4!

THANK YOU, LORD, FOR ALL THE BEAUTY AND ALL THE SPLENDOR. THANK YOU LORD FOR BREATH AND FOR

Life!

You knew then, didn't you?

No, I only suspected, Pops. I still had hope. I thought Henry might pull some miracle cure at the last minute. I really did feel that way until I left Duke and came back to Stuart. They teach you about acceptance in your program, Pops. You should know. Acceptance can come in stages. At least it did for me. It was incremental.

You just wanted to be home in the end, didn't you?

In the end there was nothing the chemo could do for me except make me sick, and there really wasn't anything Duke could do for me either. As you would say, it wasn't in the cards. I'm glad I didn't go in the hospital though, Pops, and I'm glad you and mom got me to the hospice residence. You wondered if I could hear you when I was sedated at the residence? I heard you and I heard Mom. I heard Courtney and my siblings. I heard all the voices even though I could no longer talk. It was as if I were eavesdropping on life, as if I wasn't really a part of it any more, just a member of some audience and then the curtain came down.

That's what the Hospice folks told us that at the end the dying hear the voices of their loves ones.

Your world constricts when you are dying, Pops, it gets smaller. At the end I wanted to be home. It was a reversal.

When you are little you want to cross the street, then when you are older you ride a bike a half mile and your world expands. Then you learn to drive a car and the world seems enormous. But for me, everything reversed in the end, my world grew smaller every day until it was confined to one bed in the bedroom at the Hospice residence with all my family members circled around me, loving me, but incapable of preventing the inevitable. It reminded me of the ending of a Dickens character, the family gathered around at the end. I never really got into Dickens though.

You sort of snuck away on us, Taylor.

I left when everyone was asleep, Pops. That seemed the most appropriate time. Everyone who mattered had said goodbye. Pick up my volume of Emily Dickinson, Pops, you know the poem. Read it, Pops. Read the first verse.

"Because I could not stop for Death;

He kindly stopped for me;

The Carriage held but just Ourselves

And Immortality."

* * *

I found the origin of John Gunther's title for his memoir of his son.

I never read it, Pops. I wanted a Hollywood ending. But where does he take the title?

John Donne. Holy Sonnets.

"Death be not proud, though some have called thee

Mighty and dreadful, for thou are not so;

For those whom thou think'st dost overthrow

240

Die not, poor Death, nor yet canst thou kill me."

Sounds like the spirit or the soul to me, Pops. Death can't kill the soul. He can only release it.

That's interesting, Taylor, but I think I need to call it a night. I'm a bit tired tonight.

Sleep well, Pops, but don't take any carriage rides for a while. This place is pretty crowded already.

19th Birthday

So do you remember your 19th birthday?

As well as most dead girls, I guess. It was more of a "deathday" than a birthday, Pops. I mean, let's face, there wasn't any cake and ice-cream and I was a pile of ashes in a canister. It's kind of hard to enjoy a birthday from that perspective.

Well, you died so late in November and we had you cremated. Are you sorry we didn't bury you?

Heck no, dust to dust and all of that. Fine with me. Courtney told me that when you go, Pops, you want be cremated and your ashes mixed in with the sand in the big butt can at your twelve-step group.

Yes.

I thought that was pretty funny.

Courtney didn't care for it.

No, not my serious sister, but she did a great job with my ceremony. So did mom at my funeral.

I always thought your mom did a great job at the funeral, Taylor. Better than I ever could have done.

She really did, but I liked the boat ceremony best, Pops. On the boat, a mile from the beach, letting my ashes float out to sea. And the roses and the pictures in the water.

Just one, your commencement photograph.

Well that's fine, Pops. Death really was a new beginning. Jeff wasn't there though; he was up in North Carolina.

He died shortly after that in that car accident. Like the dream you once had about him. So sad. Unbelievable. Courtney played your favorite songs. She had a mix. There were songs by Fleetwood Mac, of course, and Billy Joel and Lauryn Hill as well as "Tequila Sunrise" and "Sister Golden Hair Surprise."

That's what I always sang to Courtney, "Sister Golden Hair Surprise," it was the perfect song for her. I like it that Courtney ended the music with "When Doves Cry," by Prince. I thought that was cool.

I remember how determined you were to give Courtney a birthday gift on November 20th, her 21st birthday. You were about to get a spinal tap and all you could think about was your sister's birthday. I still hear the anguish of your cries when you got that spinal tap.

Well, it smarted quite a bit, Pops. Spinal taps aren't for the squeamish. Courtney was my sister, Pops, but she was also my dearest friend. I'm so glad I didn't die on Courtney's birthday, Pops. That would have been the worst thing possible for her. I could have died on the 27th or 28th but I had business to finish with Karly because we had a falling out.

Karly drove from Orlando to be with you at the end. The hospice folks told us that patients try to resolve issues before they pass on.

You and Courtney were an "and," Taylor, and now the "and" is gone. It is no longer Courtney and Taylor, Courtney and Taylor.

I don't know, Pops. Maybe it is, in a way. You know from the boat, you could see the shore and Bathtub Beach and Sailfish Point. That's where Courtney met her husband. What's he like?

You'd like him, Taylor. He's brilliant but sometimes absent-minded.

Sounds like you, Pops, except for the brilliant part.

You're cute.

I know it. You've got enough pictures on the wall to prove it, Pops. Damn beautiful girl wasn't I?

Yes, Taylor, in more ways than one.

I even have a picture of you lovingly holding Rhett.

Burn that photo, Pops. I have a reputation to hold up.

Chapter Forty-Nine: Ed Bradley

You never watched the program a second time, did you, Pops?

No, but I have it on tape. Several people gave me tapes of the 60 Minutes *show. April 2002, Desperately Fighting Cancer. You know I can Google Taylor Black* 60 Minutes, *Brain Cancer and you come right up.*

I guess the program will always be there. Ed Bradley sent you an email, didn't he, Pops? Just a short little email that you keep in the desk drawer with copies of my journals. Courtney has the originals of my journals.

Courtney is the historian now; she has an M.A. in history.

You never were a big fan of televising everything.

No, but I thought the attention would get you the best care. It was surreal to watch you on the program after you had passed on. You talked so calmly about death. I thought you were humble and Dr. Henry Friedman arrogant. You looked radiant.

Type out the transcript excerpts, Pops. I'll wait.

60 Minutes: April 7, 2002

Ed Bradley (voiceover): *Taylor Black, a seventeen-year-old high school senior from Florida has a rare and fast growing brain tumor which was diagnosed a year and a half ago after she collapsed in the shower.*

Taylor: *When I got the results that I had a brain tumor and everything it just didn't seem real, because you see the—you think you're invincible when you're this young. You're like "what could happen to me? What could possibly happen to me?" But it is happening to me, so I have to deal with it.*

There was a good deal of footage of Taylor with the family, especially her mom, and with Henry Friedman, and Bradley did a voiceover.

Bradley (voiceover): *We first met Taylor Black 15 months ago. She had just started being treated by Henry Friedman after leaving her original oncologist who told her that the cancer was too far advanced and that nothing could be done to save her. When she was diagnosed, she was told by her doctors that she had only six months to live.*

I certainly don't remember that discussion with any of Taylor's doctors. And the 15 months was closer to 14 months, but, what the heck, it was broadcast journalism so perhaps it was close enough. Dr. Henry Friedman then gave a voiceover.

Friedman: *Surprise, she's still here. And we're going to try to make that continue because the goal is not just a few months. The goal is to cure her which is still very possible.*

Taylor: *He is the ideal doctor for me. He's got a lot of hope.*

(Footage of Henry Friedman with the Black family, Taylor undergoing radiation treatment at Shands Hospital at the University of Florida)

Bradley (voiceover): *But Dr. Friedman's 2,000 patients don't need proof, especially the ones who are sicker than Taylor Black. Her type of cancer cannot be treated with monoclonal antibody therapy, so instead she has had two brain surgeries and undergone multiple rounds of chemotherapy with two different drugs. While the treatments seem to be slowing the growth of the tumor, Dr. Friedman added another weapon last April in hopes of destroying her cancer: high beam radiation of Taylor's brain and spine. It has caused her to lose her hair.*

Actually she lost her hair with the first rounds of chemotherapy.

Taylor (voiceover): *I had long hair, and then it just started falling out in big clumps.*

(Footage of Taylor putting on a wig).

Bradley (voiceover): *The ordeal has been intense and painful. Some people say that you* (Speaking on camera to Taylor) *you have to go to hell first.*

Taylor: *Pretty much.*

Bradley: *So you never reached a point where you said, "I just can't take this anymore?"*

Taylor: *Oh yeah, I did. I just wanted to scream and cry, but I have to take it. You know. I just have to get through it.*

Bradley: *You must have thought about the possibility that you won't beat it.*

Taylor: *Yeah, I have thought about that, definitely. I—it's a very real possibility but everybody's got to die someday, and if I have to die, I have to die. I mean, I've come to grips with my own mortality now. Nobody lives forever. If go a little bit earlier than I was—thought I was going to go then I do, but at least make every day count.*

Bradley: *You're amazing.*

Taylor (smiling): *Thank you.*

The program, watched by over twenty million people, would go on to detail one last attempt by Dr. Friedman to save Taylor and then, Ed Bradley came on with the final words about my daughter.

Taylor Black went home and two weeks later she died.

* * *

They got a few things wrong, Taylor.

Yes, but they got the story right. I mean that's what the whole thing was about after all.

Ed Bradley's email the next day said, "I was touched by Taylor's strength, maturity and openness. She was truly amazing. I can't tell you how many people have stopped me today to talk about her."

Maybe I did some good in the end, Pops.

Maybe you did, Taylor, maybe you did.

Chapter Fifty: Eternal Knight

Taylor K. Black

January 11, 1983–November 29, 2001

ETERNAL KNIGHT

April 17, 2002

University of Central Florida

That is the inscription on a triangular piece of glass that rests on a small block of wood, a memento of the "Eternal Knight" ceremony in 2002 to remember the deceased students of the University of Central Florida. It was the first such ceremony and I don't know if the university continued with the ceremony or if it has become tradition. But somewhere about 2006 or 2007 I had to Super Glue eternity back together as the glass had slipped off the block.

Taylor's Aunt Barbara and grandmother Virginia showed up for the ceremony as did Taylor's friends Karly and Gia. Taylor's roommate Celia was also there and I gave her a taped copy of the *60 Minutes* program. Taylor's mother wasn't there and she did not attend another memorial for deceased children at St. Mary's Hospital at which Taylor was honored.

It wasn't in her I guess, Pops. She doesn't live in the past like you do. You're the history teacher, you live in the past. Mom lives in the present.

That's true.

* * *

They tolled the ship's bell. So John Donne, Pops. So John Donne. "Do not ask for whom the bell tolls…"

It tolls for thee.

Kind of a small audience though, Pops, considering all the kids that croaked that year.

There were more empty chairs than full ones. Most of the big wigs of the university showed up, but the audience was family and friends. As for the student body at UCF, it was just another day of classes. Death? What is that? It doesn't concern me. I am young. I am invincible. Call me back in 60 years.

That's how I felt too, Pops, before they discovered the brain tumor. You guys cried a lot at the ceremony. Truly a Kleenex moment. Tears are God's way of cleansing the soul, I think.

I gave the roses to your grandmother.

I remember that. That was a nice gesture, Pops.

The bell rang seventeen times, Taylor, but some of the deceased were actually alumni that have passed on in the last few years. I suppose they were included because it was the first year and they were just trying to catch up.

I was happy Karly and Gia were there along with Aunt Barb and Grandma. It was special that Celia came too. I really liked Celia.

She liked you too, Taylor. She told me so. She said she was thankful for having known you. That really hit me hard. That's when I started bawling.

You always were a sentimental sap, Pops.

Just like you.

Like father…Like daughter.

Sleep well, Pops. We'll chat again….

The End

An Epilogue

"Conversation in a Car" (First published in *Living with Loss* Magazine)

By Timothy W. Black

"I can't believe you saved this car," Taylor said to her father as he turned the ignition of the 1991 Tercel, the green turtle of Taylor's high school days.

"I couldn't give it up," her father smiled wistfully.

Taylor laughed. "Dad, you are the only man I ever knew who watched Oprah and cried along with the women."

"Guilty," he smiled.

"And during *It's a Wonderful Life* every year at Christmas time. You sobbed like a sissy, dad."

"You did too, Tale."

"When Clarence got his wings, sure. I couldn't help it. Boy! They've really redone East Ocean Boulevard haven't they?" She said as he turned the old car onto the main drag in Stuart.

"Four lanes, sweetheart. Only two when you were here."

"I wish we had time to go to the beach."

"At night?"

"I always liked it after twilight, dad. Just the stars and me. Too bad you don't have time."

"We can go, sweetheart."

"No, no. You have to meet mom. Some other time."

"Okay," he sighed. "Remember when you wandered away at the Statue of Liberty. I nearly had a heart attack. You were always wandering away, Taylor."

"I guess I was. I guess I never realized that they were steps in a journey. This bridge is new isn't it?"

"Yes," the father said as he crossed the span to Sewall's Point. "I forget you haven't been here in five years."

"Yes. Five years. I guess in your mind I'm still 18 and your little girl."

"Uh huh," the father smiled. "Sometimes you are much younger. In your softball uniform. You girls were so little the fathers had to pitch in the games."

"And you *beaned* me," Taylor laughed

"Wait a minute, Tale. I yelled for you to get out of the way and you just stood there and got plunked. And then you cried."

"Of course I cried. I was eight years old and my dad had just *beaned* me with a softball. That's a funny name for the ball. There was nothing *soft* about it."

"I didn't mean to bean you."

"And those other fathers yelling *child abuse* and everyone laughed. Except me. I cried."

"Okay, okay," the father said. "How many times do I have to say I'm sorry."

"Infinity," Taylor laughed.

"You and *infinity*. That was your favorite word as a child. *Infinity*."

"I love you *infinity*."

"Yes, you always said that."

"I always meant it, dad. So my dear sister Courtney told you I smoked pot before school huh?"

"Yes. I never knew that."

"Some things are best kept from parents."

"But why?"

"Dad, it was *high* school. It was the only way to get through high school. *High.* Get it?"

"Yeah...Ha ha."

"Bad joke. C'mon, dad. I learned them from you." She began to sing. "I guess it doesn't matter anymore..."

"Buddy Holly?"

"Sure. You always played Buddy Holly on I 95 those summers we went to Nana's. And Sergeant Pepper and the Mamas and Papas. You indoctrinated us, dad."

"I corrupted you?"

"We didn't see it like that."

"Is that why you started smoking pot, Tale?"

"Geez, dad. In the end it kept me from barfing...." she sang again. "I guess it doesn't matter anymore."

"Hmmm. Pot? Is that why you never rode to school with your older sister?"

"Courtney? She was a goody two shoes. She never did anything in high school except forge notes for other kids."

"Yes, she told me that."

"When?"

"Last year."

"After the statute of limitations had run out. Watch your speed in Sewall's Point, the place always was a speed trap."

"I know."

"I always felt like I was in Courtney's shadow with you, dad. She graduated from high school with an A.A. degree from junior college. I could have done that too."

"Yes, I think you could have. But you didn't apply yourself."

"You didn't apply yourself in high school either, dad."

"Who told you that?"

"Who do you think?"

"You've been talking to Nana?"

Taylor laughed. As they drove north on Sewall's Point road past the houses on the Indian River, docks lit by lanterns like so many fireflies, they slowed for the stoplight by the marina. Taylor loved to catch fireflies when she was little, the father thought.

"Remember when we rode on Frances Langford's yacht, Tale?"

"Yes. That United Way fund raiser when you and mom were still married."

"Uh huh. What was the name of that boat?"

"The Chancellor or Chancellor, something like that," Taylor said.

"Yes, that was quite a day. She was quite a lady, Tale."

"She sure is. Up on the hill to the left, dad. Isn't that the old F.I.T. dormitory?"

"Yes. It's an assisted living place now. The rest of F.I.T. they turned into a park."

"Didn't you teach classes there?"

"Adjunct stuff. Before you were born, sweetheart. Before the college went belly up. Now look at it," he said as he turned into an entrance to the palm tree lined park. Lights from the second floor of a two story building beckoned a stream of people from their parked cars. Some of those people meandered about the second floor veranda until dimming lights, like a theater cue, invited them inside to their seats lined row upon row in front of a slide screen.

"I'm glad you came, dad," Taylor said.

"Only took five years."

"I guess it takes longer for some, dad."

"Not your mom though."

"She's different. It's okay though. You're here."

"Uh huh."

"Go, dad. Mom's waiting for you upstairs. You're on your own from here. I'm not going up with you."

"I know. I know."

As he locked his car door he smiled at his daughter then walked from the parking lot up the stairs to the second floor of the building. His ex-wife met at him at the top of the stairs and gave him his candle. He noticed that she had been crying. He knew that throughout the world on this day, hour after hour, this ceremony was being repeated.

He took the candle from his ex-wife, gave her a hug, and began to cry. His tears dotted his "Compassionate Friends" program, but at last he was here. After five years he was here and midway through the ceremony as he watched the slide of Taylor fill the screen, his salty smile eased his sorrow.

To paraphrase the late Paul Harvey, "And that was the rest of the story."

* * *

Every year in December around the world, Compassionate Friends sponsors candlelight ceremonies to remember the children who have predeceased their parents. My heart goes out to parents who have lost a child and to their siblings as well. I like to think of those lights not as candles in the wind but as the eternal flames of memory that can never go out as long as we daydream about those children.

I would like to thank *Living with Loss* Magazine for publishing "Conversation in a Car" in 2007. I would also like to thank Beth Patterson at the Virtual Teahouse for allowing me to blog about Taylor. I would also like to thank Bette Althof for her persistence in reading all the rewrites of the memoir and for her encouragement for the project.

And I would like to thank my daughter Courtney for finding Taylor's journals. Without Taylor's journals this volume could never have been completed.

Made in the USA
Columbia, SC
18 February 2021

32512125R10162